THE
SILENT KILLERS
WITHIN

Arrest them
before they strike and
add years to your life

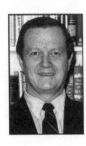

About the Author

Dr. Bruce Miller's postgraduate studies at New York University included clinical, nutrition oriented research which focused on nutrition problems of the elderly.

Dr. Miller is a member of the Linus Pauling Institute of Science Medicine, a charter member of Dr. Kenneth Cooper's Aerobics Center, a member of the International Academy of Preventive Medicine, International College of Applied Nutrition, founder of the Diet Analysis Center, and a consultant to the American Running and Fitness Association.

Dr. Miller is a Certified Nutrition Specialist and a member of the American College of Nutrition. Currently, Dr. Miller is the Director of Research for the American Academy of Nutrition. Dr. Miller lives in Dallas with his wife, Jody.

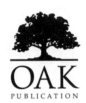

OAK PUBLICATION SDN BHD
B1-02, PJ Industrial Park, Section 13, Jalan Kemajuan,
46200 Petaling Jaya, Selangor Darul Ehsan, Malaysia.
Tel: 603-7957 6216 Fax: 603-7957 5905
E-mail: oakpublication@gmail.com
Website: www.oakpublication.com

Published by arrangement with BRUCE MILLER ENTERPRISES INC.
Copyright © 2008 by Bruce Miller

First published in Malaysia 2008
ISBN 978-983-3735-13-6

Contents

Page

1

CARDIOVASCULAR DISEASES IN THE 21ST CENTURY

The Silent Killers Within

Major Forms of CVD

The Silent Killers Within

OVERVIEW

Cardiovascular disease (CVD) has two main components: diseases of the heart (cardio) and diseases of the blood vessels (vascular). CVD, therefore, is any disease of the heart or blood vessels. This includes high blood pressure (hypertension), coronary heart disease, rheumatic heart disease and stroke, among others, and can lead to organ dysfunction.

CVD has been the number one killer in the United States every year for more than a century, except during the 1918 flu pandemic. Up to the 1900s, the causes of death were largely infectious diseases.

According to the *Heart Disease and Stroke Statistics – 2007 Update* by the American Heart Association, for the year 2004:

- 79.4 million Americans have one or more forms of CVD, of whom 37.5 million are estimated to be age 65 or older.

- CVD accounted for more deaths than any other single cause or groups of causes of death in the United States.

- Nearly 2,400 Americans die of CVD each day, an average of one death every 36 seconds.

- In 2004, CVD claimed 871,500 lives compared to cancer, which claimed 550,270 lives; accidents 108,694; Alzheimer's disease 65,829; and HIV (AIDS) 12,995.

- If all forms of major CVD were eliminated, life expectancy would rise by almost seven years, and if all forms of cancer were eliminated, the gain would be three years. The probability

3

of dying from CVD is 47 percent while the chances of dying from cancer are 27 percent.

Through numerous clinical, laboratory and population studies, scientists have been able to identify certain risk factors in the development of CVD. CVD risk factors are characteristics, conditions, habits or practices that increase a person's risk of heart attack, stroke or other forms of CVD. All statistics stated below are sourced from the 2005 and 2007 Updates of *The Heart Disease and Stroke Statistics* by the American Heart Association.

The silent killers within – pre-diabetes along with diabetes, elevated cholesterol and high blood pressure – are well established risk factors of your cardiovascular health. They are silent because these diseases fall below the threshold of perceived pain. Secondly, they occur gradually over many years without any warning or symptoms until the person experiences a debilitating side effect of the disease.

THE PRE-DIABETES CONNECTION

56.5 million people are estimated to suffer from pre-diabetes or metabolic syndrome. An estimated one million adolescents aged 12-19 have pre-diabetes.

Pre-diabetes raises the risk of developing type 2 diabetes within 10 years. People with pre-diabetes have a 1.5-fold risk of CVD compared to people with normal blood glucose.

THE DIABETES CONNECTION

In 2004, diabetes killed 72,800 people in the United States. Physician-diagnosed diabetes accounted for 15.2 million American adults. About five million cases of diabetes are undiagnosed diabetes.

Diabetes-induced heart disease and stroke: At least 65 percent of people with diabetes mellitus die from some form of heart disease or stroke. Adults with diabetes have heart disease death rates about two to four times higher than adults without diabetes. The risk for stroke is two to four times higher and the risk of death from stroke is 2.8 times higher among people with diabetes.

Diabetes-induced hypertension: About 73 percent of adults with diabetes have blood pressure greater than or equal to 130/80 millimeters of mercury (mm Hg) or use prescription medications for hypertension.

Diabetes-induced blindness: Diabetic retinopathy causes 12,000 to 24,000 new cases of blindness each year, making diabetes the leading cause of new cases of blindness in adults 20-74 years of age.

Diabetes-induced amputation: In 2002, about 82,000 non-traumatic lower-limb amputations were performed in people with diabetes. More than 60 percent of non-traumatic lower-limb amputations occur in people with diabetes. The rate of amputation for people with diabetes is 10 times higher than for people without diabetes.

Diabetes-induced sexual dysfunction: Men with diabetes are twice as likely to experience erectile dysfunction than men without diabetes. Women with type 1 diabetes are twice as likely to experience prevalence of sexual dysfunction compared with women without diabetes.

Diabetes-induced kidney disease: Diabetes is the leading cause of kidney failure, accounting for 44 percent of new cases in 2002. Forty-four thousand people with end-stage renal disease were living on chronic dialysis or with a kidney transplant.

Diabetes-induced nervous system damage: About 60 to 70 percent of people have mild to severe forms of nervous system damage, such as impaired sensation or pain in the feet or hands, and other nerve problems. Almost 30 percent of people with diabetes aged 40 years or older have impaired sensation in the feet.

THE CHOLESTEROL CONNECTION

Cholesterol is an important specific high risk factor for CVD. An estimated 105.2 million adults in the United States have total blood cholesterol values of 200 mg/dL and above and about 36.6 million have levels of 240 mg/dL and above.

79.3 million have LDL cholesterol of 130 mg/dL and above and 44.1 million with HDL cholesterol of less than 40 mg/dL.

THE HIGH BLOOD PRESSURE CONNECTION

In 2004, the estimated prevalence for high blood pressure was 72 million. High blood pressure killed 54,200 people in the United States in 2004.

People with systolic BP of 160 mm Hg or higher and/or diastolic BP of 95 mm Hg or higher have a relative risk for stroke about four times greater than those with normal BP. Hypertension precedes the development of heart failure in 91 percent of cases and is associated with two to three times higher risk for developing heart failure.

Nearly one in three adults has high blood pressure. Of those with high blood pressure, 71.8 percent were aware of their condition.

It is estimated that 37.4 percent of the U.S. population aged 20 and older has pre-hypertension, with an untreated systolic pressure of 120-139 mm Hg or untreated diastolic pressure of 80-90 mm Hg.

OTHER RISK FACTORS

The following are other well-established CVD risk factors, according to the American Heart Association:

- Cigarette smoking
- Obesity
- Family history of CVD
- Sedentary lifestyle
- Aggressive response to stress ("Type A personality")
- Certain drugs
- Alcohol

Other CVD experts strongly emphasize dietary factors that contribute to the risk factors we have listed:

- Homocysteine
- Insufficient fiber in the diet, especially soluble fiber
- Excess consumption of foods high in saturated fat or cholesterol
- Excessive intake of calories
- New research now points to a lack of heart protective nutrients as an underlying cause of heart disease
- Excessive consumption of sodium

Major Forms of CVD

Here are some statistics sourced from the *Heart Disease and Stroke Statistics – 2007 Update* by the American Heart Association of the major cardiovascular diseases connected with the silent killers within you. If they are left uncontrolled, they can stealthily damage your heart, blood vessels and important organs such as the kidney, eyes, and nerves, among others.

CORONARY HEART DISEASE (CHD)

Coronary heart disease is caused by atherosclerosis, the narrowing of the coronary arteries due to a fatty buildup of plaque, which is likely to produce angina pectoris (chest pain) and heart attack (the death of muscle cells in the heart from a lack of oxygen), or both.

Coronary heart disease is the single leading cause of death in the United States today.

It is estimated that there are 15.8 million Americans with this disease. Mortality was estimated at 452,300.

CHD caused one of every five deaths in the United States in 2004. The lifetime risk of developing CHD after age 40 is 49 percent for men and 32 percent for women.

STROKE

A stroke occurs when there is a sudden loss of blood supply to a part of the brain. This results in disruption of physical or mental functions controlled by that part of the brain.

It is estimated that 5.7 million people suffered from stroke. The mortality rate is estimated at 150,100. On an average, every three to four minutes, someone in the United States dies of a stroke. When considered separately from other forms of CVD, stroke ranks number three amongst all deaths behind heart disease and cancer.

Stroke accounted for about one out of every 16 deaths in the United States. As women tend to live longer than men, more women die of stroke every year. Women accounted for 61 percent of U.S. stroke deaths in 2004.

HEART FAILURE

Heart failure accounts for 5.2 million cases in the United States. The mortality rate in 2004 is estimated at 57,700. Eighty percent of men and 70 percent of women under the age of 65 who have heart failure will die in eight years.

At age 40, the lifetime risk of developing congestive heart failure for both men and women is one in five. The lifetime risk doubles for people with blood pressures greater than 160/90 mm Hg compared to those with blood pressures of less than 140/90 mm Hg.

Given these staggering statistics, it seems apparent that emphasis needs to be placed on the prevention of CVD, perhaps even more than its cure. This is the only way the epidemic of CVD can be arrested. It is widely acknowledged that many of the risk factors mentioned above – including the "silent killers within" associated with CVD – are well within your control.

Before we look at the link between the silent killers within you and CVD, let us find out if you are at risk of CVD.

SOURCES
Heart Disease and Stroke Statistics – 2005 Update, American Heart Association
Heart Disease and Stroke Statistics – 2007 Update, American Heart Association
The American Diabetes Association website: www.diabetes.org

CARDIOVASCULAR RISK EVALUATION

2

Age
Sex
Heredity and family history
Personal history
Diabetes
Smoking
Diet
Cholesterol level
High blood pressure
Weight
Physical activity
Stress

Cardiovascular Risk Evaluation

This evaluation gives you an idea of the changes you need to make in order to reduce your risk.

To score, simply start with zero and add the numbers shown for each criterion.

1. **Age**: As you get older your arteries age.
   - 56 or older -- add 1
   - 55 or younger --- add 0

2. **Sex**: Men have a higher risk of developing cardiovascular disease than women.
   - Male -- add 1
   - Female --- add 0

3. **Heredity and family history**: The old saying, "It runs in my family" is an indicator of serious risk.
   - A close blood relative had a heart attack or stroke before age 60 -- add 12
   - A close blood relative had heart disease before age 60, but didn't have a heart attack or stroke --- add 10
   - A close blood relative had a heart attack or stroke after age 60, and before age 80 ------------------------ add 6
   - A close blood relative had a heart attack or stroke after age 80 -- add 3
   - None of the above -- add 0

4. **Personal history**: If you already have symptoms of CVD, you are at a higher risk.
   - If you had a heart attack, stroke, heart or blood vessel surgery before age 50 ------------------------------ add 20
   - If you had one or more after age 50 -------------------- add 10
   - None of the above -- add 0

13

5. **Diabetes/Pre-diabetes:** CVD is higher among diabetics.
   - If you had diabetes before age 40
     and are using insulin -- add 10
   - If you had diabetes at or over age 40
     and are using insulin or pills ---------------------------------- add 5
   - If your pre-diabetes/diabetes began after age 55
     or can be controlled by diet ------------------------------ add 3
   - None of the above --- add 0

6. **Smoking:** Smoking is bad!
   - If you smoke two or more packs a day ------------------ add 10
   - If you smoke more than one but less than two packs
     a day or quit less than a year ago ------------------------ add 6
   - If you smoke five or more cigars a day or a pipe
     regularly -- add 5
   - If you smoke less than one pack a day or
     quit smoking for over one year ------------------------------ add 3
   - If you smoke less than five cigars a day or
     don't inhale a pipe -- add 3
   - If you quit smoking over five years ago
     but less than 20 years --- add 1
   - If you never smoked or have quit for
     over 20 years --- add 0

7. **Diet**: The "richer" your diet, the greater your risk;
   eat simple food.
   - One or more servings of red meat daily,
     seven or more eggs a week, use butter,
     whole milk and cheese --- add 8
   - If you eat red meat over four times weekly,
     over four eggs weekly, use margarine, low fat milk
     and dairy products, some cheese ------------------------- add 4
   - Poultry, fish, occasional red meat, three or fewer
     eggs, skim milk --- add 0

8. **Cholesterol level:**
   - If your total cholesterol is over 240 mg/dL ------------- add 10
   - If it is between 200-239 mg/dL ------------------------------ add 5
   - If it is less than 200 mg/dL --------------------------------------- add 0

9. **High blood pressure**: This applies to your blood pressure without medication.
   - If it is 160/100 for either number ---------------------------- add 10
   - If it is 140/90 for either number ----------------------------- add 5
   - If it is below139/89 for either number --------------------- add 0

10. **Weight**: Determine your ideal weight.
    (a) Take your height in inches. Subtract 60 and multiply by five.
    (b) If you are a woman, add 100; if you are a man, add 110.
    This is your ideal weight (in pounds).
    - If you are 25 pounds over this weight -------------------- add 4
    - If you are 10 to 24 pounds over this weight ------------ add 2
    - If you are less than 10 pounds over this weight ------- add 0

11. **Physical activity**: A lack of activity contributes to heart problems.
    - If you exercise aerobically (brisk walk, jogging, cycling, racquet ball, swimming, etc.) more than 15 minutes, less than once a week ----------------------- add 4
    - If you exercise that way twice a week ------------------ add 2
    - If you exercise that way three times a week ---------- add 0

12. **Stress**: The worst stress is internally generated stress.
    - If you are frustrated while waiting in line, anxious to complete work, anxious for appointments, easily angered, often irritable ----------------------------- add 4
    - If you are simply impatient, occasionally moody, sometimes anxious -- add 2
    - If you are relatively easygoing --------------------------- add 0

Total your score and consider your cardiovascular risk.

Score	Risk
40 or more	High
20 to 39	Medium
Less than 10	Low

This test is easy, even fun to take and the lower your score, the longer you are likely to live. See where you stand and take steps to get your score into the low bracket.

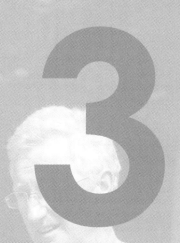

THE HEART AND CIRCULATORY SYSTEM

The Pump

Diseases Of The Heart And Blood Vessels
Stroke
High Blood Pressure
Aneurysm
Congestive Heart Failure
Angina
Heart Attack

Atherosclerosis: The Root Of Most CVD

The Pump

To understand CVD, we need to understand the mechanics of the heart and circulatory system. The heart is just one part of the cardiovascular system. It is also composed of millions of blood vessels and their billions of cells whose proper function determines cardiovascular health.

Approximately 72 times a minute, more than 100,000 times a day, the heart beats to keep circulating the five quarts of blood in the body. The heart muscle contracts, relaxes, and then contracts again, pumping two to two-and-a-half ounces of blood with each beat.

Through pencil-thick arteries, the blood flows into smaller and smaller blood vessels and then into tiny capillaries which carry it to the tissues. Oxygen and nutrients from the blood are absorbed by the tissues through the capillary walls and exchanged for carbon dioxide and cellular wastes.

Then, the oxygen-spent, nutrient-poor "used" blood is returned to the heart, passing back through the tiny capillaries, the larger blood vessels, and finally the veins. When the blood reaches the heart, it is pumped into the lungs to get rid of its carbon dioxide and to pick up a fresh supply of oxygen. Finally, it returns once again to the heart to begin the cycle all over again.

The tiny heart pump, only a little larger than a fist and weighing less than a pound, propels blood through approximately 75,000 miles of blood vessels. The process is a wondrous one, and it should continue for 70 to even 100 years.

Unfortunately, there can be problems. Something can happen that throws off the heart's rhythm – that delays or halts the heart beat – and prevents the blood from reaching its destination. The result can be an uneven beat, a rapid out-of-control beat, chest pain (angina), a heart attack, stroke, or death. Tragically, in a high percentage of cases, sudden death is the victim's first outward sign of CVD.

Diseases of the Heart and Blood Vessels

The following are a few of the more common diseases of the cardiovascular system. People with CVD may develop any of these conditions, or a combination of them.

STROKE

A stroke occurs when there is a sudden loss of blood supply to some part of the brain. This results in a disruption of physical or mental functions controlled by that part of the brain. The brain's cells can be paralyzed or killed. If they are only paralyzed, the brain cells may eventually recover and regain control of the lost functions. However, if they are killed by a lack of oxygen supply, the brain cells will never recover, and the disability usually becomes permanent.

The most common type is a thrombotic stroke. This occurs when any artery supplying blood to the brain becomes blocked. The cause is very similar to a heart attack. In fact, it could be called a "heart attack" of the brain. The artery collects cholesterol deposits over a period of time, the vessels narrow, a blood clot forms in the narrow passage, and you have a stroke. It is also called cerebral thrombosis.

HIGH BLOOD PRESSURE

High blood pressure is a modern dilemma. No one ever dies of high blood pressure. They die of other illnesses induced or made worse by high blood pressure, such as heart attack, stroke, heart failure, kidney failure, and other problems. High blood pressure also diminishes the quality of life by causing poor eyesight, morning headaches, fainting spells, depression, ringing in the ears, and others. In nearly 90 percent of the cases, high blood pressure can be controlled with diet, food supplements, and some lifestyle modifications.

ANEURYSM

An aneurysm is a localized "ballooning-out" of the wall of a blood vessel. Most incidences of aneurysm are associated with high blood pressure and atherosclerosis (loss of elasticity of the artery walls due to cholesterol deposits). The increased pressure in the blood vessel coupled with a weakened wall results in an aneurysm.

Aneurysms cause many problems by the pressure they exert on other organs of the body. Also, aneurysms may rupture and cause fatal hemorrhages.

CONGESTIVE HEART FAILURE

Congestive heart failure is the failure of the heart to maintain an adequate output of blood. Because the heart has been damaged, it is unable to pump out all of the blood that is returned to it. Consequently, blood backs up and collects in the veins and tissues, causing congestion and swelling (edema).

Heart damage may be caused by a heart attack, high blood pressure or atherosclerosis.

ANGINA

Angina is a condition in which the heart muscles receive an insufficient blood supply, resulting in chest pain and frequent pain in the left arm and shoulder. Angina is a common result of our old friend, atherosclerosis in the coronary arteries, and a primary symptom of heart disease. The pain of angina is caused by a temporary decrease in oxygen supply to the heart. The arteries become so narrowed that even mild exertion causes pain. The exertion speeds up the heart, but not enough oxygen-rich blood can be pumped to the heart muscle to keep up with the demand.

HEART ATTACK

A heart attack, sometimes known as coronary occlusion, coronary thrombosis, or myocardial infarction, refers to the sudden death of a part of the heart muscle. A heart attack results from a blockage in one of the coronary arteries due to atherosclerosis (a build up of cholesterol in the arteries).

Normal Heart Circulation

This is a heart with normal circulation. The arrows indicate the direction of blood flow in the coronary arteries.

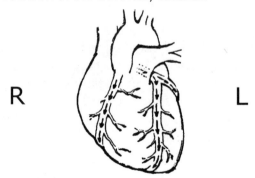

R   L

The Beginning of a Heart Attack

Cholesterol begins to silently build up in the arteries. Unless we take precautions, plaque is deposited over a period of time in these arteries. When the passageway gets narrowed, a blood clot can come along and block the blood flow to this part of the heart.

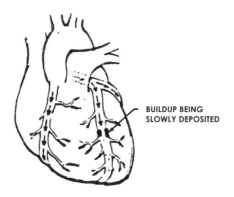

BUILDUP BEING
SLOWLY DEPOSITED

The Heart Attack

The small passageway is now totally blocked by a blood clot. This blockage hinders the blood supply to a part of the heart. Without the necessary oxygen that comes in the blood, this part of the heart becomes damaged. Depending upon the severity of the damage, disability or death can result.

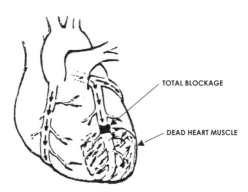

TOTAL BLOCKAGE

DEAD HEART MUSCLE

REMEMBER!

1. Blockage can develop without you being aware of it until it is too late.
2. In about 90 percent of heart attacks, a blood clot originated inside the vessel to later cause blockage.

Atherosclerosis: The Root of Most CVD

If you go back over the most common CVD, you will note that atherosclerosis is at the root of just about all of them. It's obvious that if we can prevent, halt, or even reverse the process of atherosclerosis, we can go a long way in preventing the major forms of CVD. This can be done to a great degree through proper nutrition. But first, what is atherosclerosis?

Atherosclerosis begins with a tiny bit of cellular damage to the lining of the artery wall. Many believe this initial damage is caused by an oxidant particle. During normal body function, a lot of oxygen is consumed. During this oxygen metabolism, "wild" oxygen particles called free radicals are produced. These can damage cells. We are also inundated with oxidant particles in our environment. Cigarette smoke, polluted air, and herbicides are loaded with them, as are a number of other air and water pollutants. This free radical problem has resulted in an explosion of studies on nutrients called antioxidants. These special nutrients have the ability to neutralize or block the attack of these free radicals.

After the initial damage caused by free radicals, a fatty streak appears on the lining of the artery. This can occur in someone as young as 11 years of age. As time passes, deposits of cholesterol, fibrin (a blood clotting material), calcium, and cellular debris accumulate in and on the artery. As the artery wall becomes thick and hard from this buildup, the artery narrows and loses its ability to contract and expand. The narrowing of the artery wall and loss of elasticity reduce blood flow. All of these can set you up for high blood pressure, aneurysm, congestive heart failure and angina.

The biggest danger of atherosclerosis is that a blood clot may form and completely block the already narrowed artery. When this happens, the blood flow through that artery is shut off.

When the clot is in a heart vessel, you have a heart attack. If the blockage is in a vessel that supplies the brain, you have a stroke. Can you see now why it's so important to prevent, stop, or even reverse atherosclerosis? It is at the root of most CVD.

Atherosclerosis is a silent, symptom-less disease, and a person might not be aware of a problem until something dramatic happens... such as a heart attack or a stroke. It is silent but often deadly.

Scientists still do not completely understand all the causes and processes that produce atherosclerosis, but they have learned enough to tell us how to prevent it from forming – to stop its growth – and in many cases actually reverse some of the damage. We do know for sure that eating foods high in saturated fats and cholesterol will contribute greatly to this problem.

Authorities now recommend eating foods low in cholesterol and saturated fats, and consuming a diet high in soluble fiber and certain other nutrients called antioxidants. Diet has become the primary means in helping to impede the atherosclerotic process and thus, greatly lower the risk of heart attack, stroke and other forms of CVD.

THE PRE-DIABETES CONNECTION

Overview

America is in the midst of an enormous, silent epidemic that can ruin your quality of life and also be deadly. The epidemic is called pre-diabetes, a condition of high insulin levels, high triglycerides, low HDL (good) cholesterol, insulin resistance, a growing waistline and blood glucose levels that are higher than normal but not high enough to be diagnosed as diabetes. You are in the gray zone between "normal" and "diabetic."

This condition precedes diabetes and was formerly described by a number of names such as metabolic syndrome (Syndrome X, insulin resistance syndrome), impaired glucose tolerance or impaired fasting glucose. The American Diabetes Association has officially adopted the term pre-diabetes "as a wake-up call." The other names did not seem dramatic enough to capture the essence of just how serious this problem can be. The term is not applicable to type 1 diabetes.

Although it is not as severe as diabetes, it is a condition not to be ignored, as high levels of blood glucose can sharply raise your risk of developing type 2 diabetes within 10 years, according to scientific studies. It also raises the risk of heart attack or stroke by 50 percent. Pre-diabetes is far easier to turn around in the early stages than diabetes.

Pre-diabetes is like the warning light that starts to blink when your car is about to run out of gas. Symptoms of pre-diabetes develop so gradually that most people affected by this medical condition often don't recognize it. The damage to your vital organs such as your heart, kidney, arteries, nerves and eyes are already taking place at this stage because of the high insulin level in the blood caused by your cells being insensitive to insulin. Catching the condition before it turns into full blown diabetes can be a lifesaver.

Here are three powerful statements from prominent scientists about pre-diabetes:

"People should take pre-diabetes seriously. Prevention of diabetes is possible," says Dr. Christopher Saudek, Past President of the American Diabetes Association and Professor of Medicine at Johns Hopkins University.

Dr. Francine Kaufman of the American Diabetes Association aptly says: "If you have pre-diabetes, you need to know about it, so you can learn about the high risk of getting diabetes and the steps you can take to prevent it. If you already have diabetes, you need to be treated early to prevent complications."

According to the Secretary of the US Department of Health and Human Services, Tommy G. Thompson, "The good news is if you have pre-diabetes, you can do something about it. We want people to know that pre-diabetes is a serious condition that can be reversed or alleviated with modest changes in their daily routines such as eating fewer calories and walking regularly for exercise."

What is the Cause of Pre-diabetes?

Pre-diabetes is the result of a collision between evolutionary genetics and modern living in which food is overabundant and physical exertion is only optional. Our bodies have not had time to adjust to our infatuation for processed carbohydrates laden with fat and sugar and our lack of physical activity. As a result, our blood sugar control system is not functioning well at all. Our cells become insulin resistant and blood sugar goes up. We are fatigued, suffer weight gain, and have great difficulty in losing weight.

In the early 1900s however, pre-diabetes and diabetes were hardly prevalent as the carbohydrates consumed by man consisted mainly of unprocessed grains and cereals, unrefined flour and unrefined molasses, compared to the refined packaged and fast food we see currently lining our supermarkets and hypermarkets. Besides, they were also more physically active.

A NOTE ON NUMBERS

Mmol/L stands for millimoles/liter and is the world standard unit for measuring glucose in blood while in the United States, the traditional unit for measuring blood glucose is mg/dL (milligrams/deciliter). If you wish to convert mg/dL of glucose to mmol/L, just divide the figure by 18.

NORMAL BLOOD GLUCOSE/INSULIN METABOLISM

In a healthy person, the carbohydrates eaten are broken down through the digestive process and converted into glucose. Glucose is then absorbed into the bloodstream. As blood glucose rises after a meal, a signal goes to the pancreas to release insulin. The hormone insulin produced in the beta cells of your pancreas moves the glucose from the bloodstream into the cells for energy production. As the blood sugar drops, insulin shuts off until it is needed again. However, if for some reason your blood sugar level gets too low, the alpha cells in your pancreas quickly secrete a hormone called glucagons, which quickly brings up your sugar level up again.

Any excess glucose in the blood is converted into a starch called glycogen and stored in the muscle and liver cells for future use. Once these stores are full, the excess glucose is converted into fats called triglycerides, which are then carried in the bloodstream to your fatty tissues where it will be deposited as fat.

In people with normal insulin metabolism, the cells are not resistant or insensitive to insulin, and as such only a small amount of insulin is required to keep the glucose level in the blood at a healthy level.

As there is no excess insulin circulating in the blood, people in this category do not have to battle with their weight problem. As their blood sugar is generally more stable, they do not have strong cravings, especially for processed carbohydrates, as compared to those whose bodies' cells are insulin resistant.

PRE-DIABETES

What happens if the cells refuse to let insulin shuttle the glucose into the cell? This is called insulin resistance. This resistance causes glucose to remain high in the bloodstream.

In order to bring down the high glucose level in the blood, the pancreas has to keep pumping out higher and higher amounts of insulin to overcome the resistance of the cells. Ultimately, by sheer force, insulin gets the glucose into the cells. Glucose levels drop but the bloodstream is elevated with insulin. The excessive insulin floating in your bloodstream is as damaging as high blood glucose. You have now increased your risk of cardiovascular problems like heart attack or stroke.

At this stage, there is nothing wrong with your pancreas except that your cells are insensitive to insulin. This is the heart of pre-diabetes. Your glucose level is not high enough to be classified as diabetes, so you are not diagnosed with type 2 diabetes. Most people who develop type 2 diabetes have pre-diabetes first.

Research indicates that each year between four and nine percent of people with pre-diabetes go on to develop type 2 diabetes. Pre-diabetics have one and a half times the risk of developing cardiovascular disease, compared to those who have normal glucose levels.

TYPE 2 DIABETES

If you do not take preventive measures to bring down your blood sugar level close to normal, over time, your pancreas will become totally overworked and cannot produce enough insulin to overcome insulin resistance. This causes abnormally high blood sugar levels and the excess sugar spills over into your urine and passes out of the body. You are now on the road to type 2 diabetes.

At this stage, the high sugar levels will damage your nerves and blood vessels, leading to long-term complications.

I DON'T HAVE TYPE 2 DIABETES, SO WHAT IS THE BIG DEAL?

This is my big concern. The so-called normal fasting blood glucose is from 70-100 mg/dL (formerly 70-110 mg/dL). You are not declared "diabetic" until your blood sugar goes above 125 mg/dL. What in the world is going on in your body when your fasting sugar is between 100 and 125 mg/dL? You can't be a little pregnant, but you can have a little diabetes.

The big deal is that the high insulin levels floating in your blood is silently injuring your health for several reasons:

- They cause the liver to increase the production of triglycerides (a kind of blood fat). High levels of triglycerides in the blood make your blood thick and sticky, increasing your risk of blood clots.

- They can cause HDL – the good cholesterol – to go down. The combination of high triglycerides and low HDL cholesterol is detrimental to your heart.

- High insulin in the blood causes the liver to manufacture more of the "bad" (LDL) cholesterol.

- They can promote storage of excess fat, especially in the abdominal area.

- They can cause your blood pressure to rise.

- They cause the buildup of plaque in your artery walls, increasing your risk of atherosclerosis (hardening of the arteries).

- They can cause slow clearing of blood fats after a meal.

- They stimulate hunger pangs, especially for carbohydrates.

- They slow down the ability of the body to break up blood clots.

With blood sugar levels between 100 and 125 mg/dL, you are slowly increasing your risk of heart disease and may ultimately go down the road to full blown diabetes.

How Do I Know If I Have Pre-diabetes?

You may have pre-diabetes if you have four or more of the following six factors:

OVERWEIGHT OR OBESE

Recent research has clearly identified that pre-diabetes is caused by insulin resistance, meaning that your body cells no longer respond to insulin's command. If you have insulin resistance, dieting and exercise may not help you lose weight permanently – no matter how hard you try. Eighty percent of those with insulin resistance are overweight. They have excess weight around the waist (more than 35.5 inches for men and 31.5 inches for women).

Insulin resistance and high levels of insulin in the blood contribute to weight gain in five different ways:

- Encourage the storage of fats as less glucose is converted into energy. Insulin has often been called "the fat-producing hormone." The excess fats normally accumulate in the abdominal area and the trunk.

- Strong craving occurs, as does excessive eating, especially for sugar and refined carbohydrates (the main source of glucose) because the body isn't efficiently converting it to energy.

- It is difficult for sugar to enter the muscle, fat and liver cells, causing high levels of sugar to be built up in the blood. The cells become starved for energy and fatigue occurs.

- Eating binges occur.

- As your cells continue to be less sensitive to insulin and you continue to gain more weight, your body further loses its ability to process foods properly, causing even more weight gain.

SEDENTARY LIFESTYLE

A sedentary life can lead to obesity. Obesity is the result of an imbalance between energy intake and energy output. Obesity does not cause insulin resistance but if you are genetically more insulin resistant, obesity does make insulin resistance worse. The more insulin resistant you become, the more insulin your pancreas secretes. Your risk of developing pre-diabetes is greater as your blood insulin level goes higher.

FASTING SUGAR SLIGHTLY HIGH (BETWEEN 100 and 125 mg/dL)

When your fasting blood sugar level is above 100 mg/dL, it tells us that your insulin is incapable of controlling your blood sugar levels within the normal range. This is a clear indicator that you are developing insulin resistance and increases your risk of pre-diabetes.

LOW HDL CHOLESTEROL BELOW 40 mg/dL FOR MEN
AND BELOW 60 mg/dL FOR WOMEN

Elevated insulin in pre-diabetics will cause the "good" HDL cholesterol to go down and increase your risk of heart disease. HDL cholesterol carries cholesterol away from the arteries back to the liver, where it is prepared for elimination through the bile. The higher your HDL, the more cholesterol can be eliminated from your body, and the lower your risk of heart disease.

HIGH TRIGLYCERIDES OVER 130 mg/dL

Triglycerides are the storage form of fat in the body. They are derived primarily from the fats you eat or excess calories from alcohol or carbohydrates.

A high level of triglycerides in the blood is often accompanied by elevated total cholesterol, LDL cholesterol and low levels of HDL. Triglycerides in large amounts thicken your blood, clog your blood vessels and form clots. When there is a blockage in the artery feeding blood to your heart, you may suffer a heart attack.

HIGH BLOOD PRESSURE OF 130/85 OR ABOVE

Blood pressure is read as two numbers: systolic and diastolic. Systolic pressure is generated when your heart muscle contracts and forcefully sends the blood through the arteries. The diastolic pressure is the remaining pressure in the arteries when the heart is refilling and getting ready to beat again. If your systolic pressure is 130 and your diastolic is 85, it would be written as 130/85 or described as "one-thirty over eighty-five."

Excess insulin in a pre-diabetic can narrow the arteries, making it difficult for blood to flow through, thereby pushing up your blood pressure. Silently and relentlessly, high blood pressure wears out and ages the large and small arteries of your body; your body vessels actually degenerate. The heart grows in size to try to push the blood against the pressure, and at the same time it begins to tire out – congestive heart failure is likely to occur. Your kidneys are scarring and shrinking. The retina of your eyes may become damaged, leading to loss of sight. Fatty deposits are increasing on the artery walls. High blood pressure is a prime risk factor for heart attacks.

Some researchers add two more elements to the above six because they are nearly always present.

GENETIC

Almost 80 percent of pre-diabetics have a family history of type 2 diabetes.

HIGH CONSUMPTION OF PROCESSED CARBOHYDRATES

The main culprit of pre-diabetes is carbohydrate as it has a direct impact on sugar level in the blood – unlike fats and protein. As we cannot predict how a carbohydrate behaves in the body just by looking at the sugar or starch content, researchers have developed an index called the Glycemic Index (GI) to rank carbohydrate foods. It indicates how fast the carbohydrate of a particular food is converted into glucose in the bloodstream. High GI food causes blood glucose to rise quickly, while low GI foods cause a steady rise. As a guideline, think of the GI as a measure of starchiness instead of sweetness.

Generally, foods that undergo the least processing have a low GI. Raw foods have lower GI values than cooked food. The majority of Americans consume a diet of high in GI foods. More than 45 percent of their calories come from breads, sugared drinks, cookies, and other highly processed commercial products.

What Should I Do if I Am Diagnosed with Pre-diabetes?

Follow the simple six step plan below. Can you reverse pre-diabetes with the plan? The answer is a definite "yes!" Can you reverse type 2 diabetes? The answer is a definite "maybe." It depends on how far your disease has progressed.

THIS IS THE SIX-STEP PLAN

Step 1: Test your blood glucose

First of all, see your doctor to get a good physical examination to discover your blood glucose numbers. Your doctor can diagnose whether you have pre-diabetes by testing your:

Fasting Blood Glucose (Blood Sugar) Level

This is done by taking a sample in the morning, after fasting for at least 12 hours or more the night before. Plain water is allowed during the fast.

The Expert Committee on the Diagnosis and Classification of Diabetes Mellitus has recently lowered the reading for pre-diabetes from 110 mg/dL to 100 mg/dL. The new cut off is expected to increase the number of people afflicted with pre-diabetes. For guidelines, see Table 1.

Table1: Fasting blood glucose guideline

Reading (mg/dL)	Diagnosis
From 70 to 100	Normal glucose tolerance
Above 100 to 125	Pre-diabetes
Above 125	Diabetes

Oral Glucose Tolerance Test (OGTT)

This test is to determine the ability of the body to handle excess sugar present after drinking a high dose of glucose solution. After fasting the night before, your doctor will take your fasting blood sugar. Following this, you will be given 75 grams of glucose with 200-300 ml of water.

For the next two hours, half hourly blood samples will be taken and the values plotted on a glucose tolerance graph, where any deviation from the normal can be determined. For guidelines, see Table 2.

Table 2: Guideline of OGTT for men and non-pregnant women after a 75-gram glucose drink

2-Hour Plasma Glucose Result (mg/dL)	Diagnosis
Below 140	Normal
From 140 to 200	Pre-diabetes (impaired glucose tolerance)
Above 200	Diabetes*

*Confirmed by repeating the test on a different day.

Step 2: Lose weight

The underlining cause of weight gain especially around the abdominal area is insulin resistance. Obesity does not cause insulin resistance. It is insulin resistance that causes obesity. When your cells are resistant to insulin, it is very difficult to lose weight permanently as high levels of insulin in the blood can promote storage of excess fat. The more weight you put on, the more insulin resistance you develop. Slimming down is one way to help lower insulin level by making your insulin more effective, thus reducing your risk of pre-diabetes.

A recent research shows that being overweight appeared to be more harmful than being inactive. Thin people who are inactive had a lower risk than active women who are overweight. However, thin people who do not exercise are also at an increased risk of developing heart disease. The truth of the matter is, to reduce your risk of cardiovascular disease; you must maintain a normal weight and remain physically active. Overweight or inactivity is an independent risk factor of heart disease.

Weight loss will help you control your sugar levels better, help lower your blood pressure, and make it easier for you to exercise, which in itself will reduce your insulin resistance.

The best way to lose weight is to eat a little less and exercise a little more. Avoiding processed carbohydrate and fatty foods is one effective way of keeping your weight down. According to the Diabetes Prevention Program, an overweight individual who loses five to seven percent of his weight accompanied by 30 minutes of exercise, five times a week may help normalize blood sugar.

The American Diabetic Association also recommends:

- Anyone who is overweight and aged 45 or older should be tested for pre-diabetes.

- Those aged 45 or older whose weight falls within healthy levels should ask their doctor about testing for pre-diabetes.

- People who are overweight but younger than 45, may seek testing for pre-diabetes if other risk factors such as high triglycerides, low HDL cholesterol, high blood pressure and elevated sugar in the blood are present.

There are two popular measurements to determine whether you are obese or overweight:

Body Mass Index (BMI): This index is used to determine if your body weight is appropriate for your height. The disadvantage of this measurement is that it does not take into account how muscular you are or where the fat is located in your body. To calculate your BMI, divide your weight by your height squared.

Body Mass Index

Underweight :	<18.5
Normal:	18.5 - 24.9
Overweight:	25 - 29.9
Obesity:	30 - 39.9
Extreme obesity:	>40

Waist measurement: It measures how much intra-abdominal fat – the fat that is wrapped around your intestine and other abdominal organs – you have. The bigger your waist, the more intra-abdominal fat you have. Your waist circumference is the best indicator of how much fat is in your abdomen.

Men are often apple-shaped with fat most likely found around the tummy than the bum; women are more pear-shaped, where the bum is wide and the hip is narrow.

The World Health Organization states that a man is obese if his waist circumference is more than 35.5 inches; a woman is considered obese if hers exceeds 31.5 inches.

Step 3: Eat better

- As carbohydrates have a direct impact on blood glucose in the blood than fats and proteins, your diet should consist of unrefined carbohydrates. "Nature-made" carbohydrates are better than "man-made" carbohydrates. Products made from grains (corn) and tubers (potatoes), which grow above the ground, have the highest glycemic index.

  Thus, to keep your insulin and sugar at a healthy level, limit your intake of refined carbohydrates found mainly in commercially processed foods such as breads, packaged cereals, sweet cakes, biscuits, cookies, chips, candies, chocolate, ice cream, packaged snack foods and instant noodles. For more information on the impact of carbohydrates on your blood sugar, I recommend *The Glucose Revolution* by Dr. Jennie Miller.

  Along with unrefined carbohydrates, add plant foods to your daily meal. Non-starchy vegetables like asparagus, bok choy, broccoli, cabbage, celery, lettuce, mushroom, green pepper, spinach and tomatoes, as well as nuts, seeds, grains, legumes and fruits that contain fibers slow down the absorption of sugar. These foods all contain a variety of antioxidants to fight free radicals, besides containing vital vitamins and enzymes that keep us healthy.

- Restrict foods that contain high levels of saturated fats and cholesterol such as fatty meat, dairy products, chicken skin, coconut oil, lard, whole milk, organ meats (liver, kidney and brains, etc.) and other high cholesterol foods.

- Restrict salty foods. They are bad for your blood pressure.

- Avoid foods and oils containing trans fatty acids, a type of fat produced by the industrial treatment of oils to make them solid at room temperature. This gives products a long shelf life. Trans fatty acids are worse than saturated fats. Saturated fats raise your bad cholesterol (LDL) while leaving your good cholesterol (HDL) unaffected, but trans fatty acids not only increase the "bad" cholesterol and triglycerides, but also decrease HDL – the "good" cholesterol – all risks factors for heart disease.

Most commercially prepared foods are high in trans fatty acids. The top 10 trans fatty acid foods are: margarine, packaged foods, soups, fast foods, frozen foods, baked foods, chips and crackers, breakfast foods (cereal and energy bars), cookies and candy, toppings and dips.

- Reduce your habit of drinking too much carbonated drinks, juice concentrates and syrups that contain too much sugar.

- Eat cold water fish such as salmon and cod rich in omega-3 fatty acids made up essentially of eicosapentaenoic acid (EPA) and docosahexaenoic acid (DHA), which are good for your heart. If you find difficulty eating fish, take an EPA/DHA food supplement.

- Read labels before buying any product. Words ending in "ose" like sucrose, lactose, maltose, fructose, glucose and dextrose, as well as honey and molasses, are all forms of sugar.

- Eat small frequent meals throughout the day to maintain proper sugar levels. Cut out snacking. Eating like a deer is better than eating like a bear.

- Avoid all processed low-fat foods. In order to compensate for the loss in fat, food manufacturers add more processed carbohydrates.

- Take high quality proteins everyday such as lean meat (free range, if possible), eggs, beans and nuts like walnuts, pecans, pistachios, almonds and hazelnuts that contain omega-3 fatty

44

acids. Avoid nuts that contain sugar coating, coloring and preservatives.

- Drink eight glasses of purified water everyday. Avoid water sold in plastic containers as they may contain Bisphenol A (BPA), which is toxic to your body. Don't reuse plastic bottles as they may be contaminated with bacteria.

- Avoid foods cooked at high temperatures or charred food; instead steam, poach, stew or bake your food as much as possible. Use herbs and natural spices to boost the taste of your meals.

- Keep away from genetically modified (GM) foods. In the United States, GM foods are treated like natural foods and it is not compulsory for it to appear on food labels. Most berries, corn, soybean, wheat, rice, tomatoes, sports drinks, baby food, frozen dinners, cereal and hamburger buns are just some examples of GM foods. You can find a comprehensive list of GM and non-GM foods at www.truefoodnow.org.

Step 4: Lead a healthy lifestyle

- **Smoking or drinking**
  Don't drink or smoke. Drinking alcohol can increase your triglycerides level, which is a high risk factor tor heart disease. Smokers also have higher triglycerides and lower HDL cholesterol. There is a strong link between cigarette and heart disease.

- **Stress**
  Manage your stress level as it may play a role in causing heart disease. Stress increases your nutritional needs. It depletes your store of magnesium and antioxidant vitamins B, C and E, which

play an important part in your health.

Learn to manage stress. Take control of your stress by treating it as a challenge and not a threat. Resist thoughts like jumping to negative conclusions or negative generalizations. Just say "no" to stress if you see one coming. Be happy and learn to say "no." Simplify your life.

If you are under stress, get support from friends, family members and trusted colleagues instead of letting the stress "eat" you up. Learn how to release your stress.

One of the simplest ways is to stop what you are doing and take a few minutes to breathe deeply. Changing your lifestyle, learning how to relax, and eating well are good ways to handle stress. Count your blessings. Be a good cheer to people around you, in your home and workplace.

- **Exercise**

  Get more exercise. Diet alone does not control insulin and sugar levels nearly as well as diet plus exercise and weight control.

  Exercise can help our body's cells be more sensitive to insulin. When you are exercising, your muscles can extract glucose from the bloodstream without the assistance of insulin. Exercise, therefore, makes blood glucose drop by increasing the rate at which muscles take up glucose. This is a key reason for diabetics to exercise.

  Doing moderate exercise three times a week can help reduce your risk of heart disease, as it helps burn extra calories, and raises your HDL cholesterol while lowering your bad cholesterol and blood pressure, and reduces your risk for atherosclerosis. High levels of insulin prevents fat from being used as a fuel source, making it difficult for diabetics to lose weight.

  Exercise strengthens the heart, lowers the resting heart rate, improves the health of your lungs and circulatory system, as well as lowers your blood pressure.

Exercise can improve your HbA1c count. A review of several published studies on the effect of exercise on diabetes confirms that exercise is beneficial for blood glucose control. The mean HbA1c was 7.65 percent for those who exercised compared to 8.32 percent for those who did not. For more details on HbA1c, turn to page 92.

A good exercise program should focus on aerobic activities that are enjoyable and done on a regular basis like brisk walking, jogging/running, cycling, swimming, hiking, racket games, rowing and others to help increase your heartbeat – provided that you are working at 50 to 70 percent of your maximum possible effort.

It would therefore be advisable to take a reading of your blood glucose level before you begin to exercise, when you have finished and again later on.

Step 5: Take drugs

Take drugs if needed. Your blood pressure, cholesterol and triglycerides might need urgent attention. But taking medications for whatever reason is dangerous without a prescription from your doctor.

Step 6: Take food supplements

Finally, take food supplements that can help you lower your blood sugar as well as improve the sensitivity of your cells to insulin.

Supplements for Pre-diabetes

Today's approach to preventing pre-diabetes is through a combination of diet, exercise and food supplementation. The objective of any supplementation program must show the following benefits:

- Helps maintain normal sugar levels

- Helps your body be more effective in utilizing blood sugar

- Helps avoid the ravages of pre-diabetes

- Prevents sugar crashes that can lead to feelings of low energy, hunger, carbohydrate cravings and between-meal snacking

- Protects the cells and their structures from the damages caused by free radicals

- Helps reduce weight and control appetite

- Maintains long-term health and avoid the complications of chronic high sugar levels

- Treats the cause of insulin resistance itself

Aside from the above objectives, your supplementation program must also keep your triglycerides, HDL cholesterol, blood pressure and HbA1c at a healthy level. All these will help reduce your risk of heart disease, stroke and type 2 diabetes.

I consider the following supplements essential to help your body to be more sensitive to insulin (attack the problem of insulin resistance) and lower sugar in the blood to as near normal as possible in order to reduce your risk of pre-diabetes:

NUTRITIONAL SUPPLEMENTS

Alpha Lipoic Acid (ALA)

European and U.S. studies have shown ALA to be the most important antioxidant for diabetics. Antioxidant protection is especially vital for those who are pre-diabetic because they simply produce more oxidant particles. Free radicals fly around like bullets and can knock pieces of cells and damage or destroy sensitive insulin receptors (doors to the cells).

ALA offers incredible protection for insulin receptors. Here is why: It is more effective against a greater variety of free radicals than any other antioxidant. It is unique, in that, it can function in either the watery or fatty part of the cell membrane. Vitamin C and E lose their power after they neutralize oxidant particles but ALA can regenerate these vitamins back to their original forms.

A lot of ALA are found in the power generator of the cell called the mitochondria. It acts as an enzyme that helps burn sugar for energy. In fact, ALA is so efficient that it always seems to need more glucose to burn. The mitochondria use their "cell phone" to call the insulin receptor and tell it to relax a bit and let in some glucose. This request improves insulin receptor function, lowering the blood sugar level.

Zinc

Supplemental zinc is essential for those who are pre-diabetic.

Insulin is protein assembled in the beta cells of the pancreas. The inactive insulin is stored inside the beta cells in little sacks. Zinc enters the storage sacks and activates the insulin to full power. Optimal zinc is essential to energize and release insulin.

Zinc also helps with the insulin hook-up to receptors on the cells. Think of insulin as a space shuttle and the insulin receptor as a docking port on the mother ship, which is the cell. Zinc carefully guides the shuttle to the docking port with the mother ship.

Those with pre-diabetes desperately need extra zinc. The Daily Value (DV) for zinc is 15 mg, but the average American consumes only 11.6 mg per day. To make things worse, for some reason (probably genetic), a diabetic's pancreas contains only half the amount of stored zinc as compared to a normal pancreas.

Chromium

This mineral functions as the active part of a compound known as glucose tolerance factor (GTF). GTF chromium forms a tight connection between insulin and insulin receptors. This connection allows glucose to flow into the target cell. I try to use analogies to explain some of this complex stuff. Here comes one. GTF connects to the insulin receptor like a good suction cup sticking to a glass. Bad suction cup equals bad connection. Without chromium, insulin's action is blocked and blood sugar levels are elevated. In fact, the very first sign of a chromium deficiency is elevated blood sugar. Over 15 solid, controlled studies demonstrate the positive effect of chromium on impaired glucose tolerance.

Here are the great American problems. An astounding 90 percent of us consume less than the recommended amount of chromium each day. Our diet, which is high in simple sugars and refined flour (The Standard American Diet), greatly increases the need for chromium. Chromium deficiencies are common in those who are insulin resistant.

Magnesium

This is a very busy mineral. It is involved in well over 300 enzymatic reactions in the body. Enzymes are compounds that cause the biochemical reactions in our body to go to completion. Many actions in insulin carbohydrate metabolism are dependent upon magnesium containing enzymes. Thus, this mineral has a central role in all the functions of insulin. Without adequate magnesium, control of blood sugar levels is impossible.

Pre-diabetic patients routinely have low magnesium. A main reason for these low magnesium levels is that even a slight kidney damage can cause it to be lost in the urine. The American Diabetes Association sponsored a consensus panel to examine the data on magnesium and they came out with some definite answers. I quote: "In conclusion, the weight of experimental data presented to the consensus panel suggests that magnesium deficiency may play a role in insulin resistance, carbohydrate intolerance, and high blood pressure."

AYURVEDIC HERBS

Ayurvedic herbs have been used in India for centuries, for the purpose of lowering excessive sugar in the blood and improving the sensitivity of the body to insulin. Ayurvedic herbs are recently getting serious attention in the United States.

These three herbs listed below can be taken individually or combined together in one formula for its synergistic effect.

Gymnema sylvestre
The Hindus call it gumar or "sugar destroyer." Many studies in India have shown that this herb can improve glucose intolerance and enhance insulin sensitivity. It also significantly improves cholesterol and triglyceride levels. Gymnema also helps reduce the craving for sugar and refined carbohydrates.

The recommended dose by most herbalist is 400 to 600 mg, one to three times daily of an extract standardized to contain 24 percent gymnemic acids.

Bitter Melon (Momordica charantia)
It is also known as bittergourd. A few animal and preliminary human studies suggest that it may help the body to lower blood sugar level

and enhance insulin resistance. Be careful as it may lower your need for medication if you are on an anti-diabetic prescription drugs.

The recommended dosage is three times a day standardized to 7 percent bitter acids and 0.5 percent charantin. Momordicin is the substance responsible for its bitter taste.

Fenugreek (Trigonella foenum graecum)

Studies in animal and human trials have shown that fenugreek has a high fiber content that can reduce fasting blood sugar and improve glucose tolerance and serum cholesterol levels in people with diabetes. As the seeds are bitter, it is best to take it in the form of a capsule.

Most herbalists recommend a dosage of 2.5 grams (capsule) of seed powder twice a day. It is best to take an hour before your two largest meals of the day.

It is generally safe. The only common side effect is mild gastrointestinal upset when taken in high doses.

ANTIOXIDANT SUPPLEMENTS

High sugar levels in the blood contribute to the production of free radicals as oxygen loves glucose. If not neutralized by antioxidants, free radicals can cause damage in the key arteries to the heart and the brain, and can lead to heart attack and stroke respectively in people with pre-diabetes.

Vitamin C

Vitamin C is not produced in the body but must be obtained from food. It is a water soluble antioxidant and protects the watery part of the cell membrane from free radical damage.

Vitamin C works with vitamin E to prevent the oxidation of lipoprotein (such as HDL and LDL cholesterol) that can lead to heart disease. It plays a very important role in preserving the health of our cardiovascular system.

According to Dr. Matthias Rath M.D., a well known physician and scientist, pioneer in vitamin research and cellular health, and author of *Why Animals Don't Get Heart Attacks But People Do*: "Vitamin C corrects cellular imbalances caused by elevated blood sugar levels, contributes to lower insulin requirements, decreases glucose elimination in the urine and, above all, protects the artery walls."

Studies done in the United States show that vitamin C also plays a role in reducing high blood pressure. The evidence is so strong, convincing and conclusive that the US Department of Agriculture said people with borderline hypertension may benefit from a supplement of 1,000 mg a day.

Vitamin E

Its antioxidant property offers protection for pre-diabetics against coronary artery disease. It offers protection to the cell membranes. Without sufficient vitamin E in the body, lipids and protein will become defenseless against free radical attacks. The oxidative damage by free-radicals will trigger the formation of plaque. As the plaque deposits grow, the major arteries leading to the heart can become clogged or narrowed. This blocks blood flow to the heart and a heart attack occurs.

Vitamin E can render the platelets in blood circulation less sticky, to keep the blood thin and decrease the rate of blood clotting.

There is abundant scientific evidence to show that vitamin E can reduce the risk of heart disease and can even prevent a second heart attack in patients who already suffered one.

Exercise can cause an increase in free radical activity but vitamin E can protect against some of the damage caused by physical exercise.

Andreas Papas, PhD, an author with extensive experience in antioxidants and vitamin E, has this to say in his book *The Vitamin E Factor*: "Taking an antioxidant supplement is the number one practice of cardiologists as a way to prevent heart attack. Topping the list of antioxidants is vitamin E."

Coenzyme Q10

CoQ10 is made in the liver. It is found in every cell membrane in the human body. Research shows that by middle age, you could be seriously deficient in CoQ10. The most sensible thing to do is supplement your diet with CoQ10.

The heart is the tissue most sensitive to low levels of CoQ10. CoQ10 is found in the highest amounts in your mitochondria (the "energy producing factory") of your heart muscles. It provides the "spark" each cell needs to initiate energy. Without enough CoQ10 in your body, you will run out of energy. This property is especially critical for the muscles of the heart.

Low tissue and blood levels of CoQ10 have been reported in literature concerning a wide spectrum of heart and vascular problems. The list includes congestive heart failure, coronary artery disease, high blood pressure, ventricular arrhythmia and valve disease.

"I believe that cardiovascular disease may be very significantly caused by a deficiency of CoQ10," reports Dr. Karl Folkers, a biochemist at the University of Texas.

"It is unthinkable for me to practice good cardiology without the help of CoQ10. And, for the thousands of people with cardiac conditions so severe that they need a heart transplant, CoQ10 may be a suitable alternative that not only enhances the quality of life, but extends survival as well," says Stephen Sinatra, MD, FACC, cardiologist and author of *The Coenzyme Q10 Phenomenon*.

If you are on cholesterol lowering medication, I suggest you supplement your diet with CoQ10, as the medication not only blocks the production of cholesterol in the liver, but it also blocks the body's natural production of CoQ10.

It makes good sense not to wait until a heart problem occurs before we supplement our diet with CoQ10. Taking CoQ10 from mid-life onwards could have a protective effect on the mitochondria of the heart and preserve heart function.

SUMMARY

Pre-diabetes develops gradually and silently over many years without much visible symptoms. It is advisable to take action now if you have a strong family history of diabetes, high blood pressure or heart disease but you do not currently suffer from these disorders yourself.

On the other hand, if you have begun to develop excess fat especially around your waist, have hypertension, elevated triglycerides (blood fat) accompanied by low HDL cholesterol, impaired fasting glucose or impaired glucose tolerance – you are already showing signs of pre-diabetes and damage to your vital organs such as your heart, kidney, eyes and nerves may have already begun. See your doctor immediately for a diagnosis.

The recently completed Diabetes Prevention Program study gave hope to many people with pre-diabetes. The program concluded that people with pre-diabetes can prevent type 2 diabetes from developing if they make early changes to their diet and increase their level of physical activity. Their blood sugar may even return to normal range.

They also highlighted that some medications may be able to delay the development of diabetes but diet and exercise worked better. The program recommends 30 minutes a day of moderate physical exercise coupled with a 5 to 10 percent reduction in body weight may result in a 58 percent reduction in developing diabetes.

A recent study found in the *Journal of American Medical Association* reported that people with a waistline of 30 inches had a two-fold chance of developing heart attack or stroke. The Nurses Health Study, after looking at the diabetes risk of over 40,000 women, came to the conclusion that those with 35.5 inches waistline had 20 times chance of developing diabetes compared to women with a waist circumference of 28 inches.

It is important to work closely with your doctor to monitor your lipid numbers and your sugar level on a regular basis to keep pre-diabetes at bay.

If you have pre-diabetes, take action to prevent it from progressing to full blown diabetes. It is far easier to turn pre-diabetes around in the early stages. Once you have diabetes, there is very little hope of reversing it. For the rest of your life, you will have no choice but to change the way you eat and the way you live. It also means you have to be very selective in your food intake, besides having the tedious task of monitoring your blood glucose everyday. Ask a diabetic and he will tell you his misery.

My advice to you is to do everything in your power to prevent pre-diabetes from taking hold of your body. No pre-diabetes, no diabetes! I sincerely hope that you will take immediate action to see your doctor to know your status, if you have some of the symptoms of pre-diabetes.

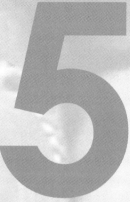

THE DIABETES CONNECTION

Understanding Diabetes

HIGH ACHIEVERS

What do all of the following famous people have in common: Thomas Edison, Ernest Hemingway, Jackie Gleason, Jackie Robinson, Elvis Presley, William Conrad, Ella Fitzgerald, Peggy Lee, Mary Tyler Moore, Thomas P. (Tip) O'Neill, Mario Puzo and Fred Silverman? Answer: They all have or have had diabetes. But consider this list carefully. They are or were among some of the highest achievers in their respective fields. Diabetes did not, and does not prevent them from living very successful lives. If you have diabetes, you can still live your life to the fullest!

The prevention of the complications of diabetes will be the main thrust of this chapter. Even if you take insulin or one of the oral drugs, statistics show you will still develop diabetic complications.

If you already have diabetes, following suggestions in this chapter will help you to avoid or lessen the complications that can destroy your quality of life.

WHAT IS DIABETES MELLITUS?

This is what the old text books used to call sugar diabetes. The name "diabetes mellitus" is from the Greek language. "Diabetes" is a term that means "to go through." That is because frequent urination is a major symptom of this disease. The word "mellitus" was added in the 17th century. It comes from the Latin word for honey. This refers to the sugar that shows up in the urine.

In fact, some early cases used to be discovered by finding ants feeding on urine passed by diabetics.

Simply put, diabetes is a disorder of the body's mechanism for utilizing sugar, or glucose, which is its basic fuel.

There are two major forms of diabetes. One is type 1, or "juvenile diabetes," because its symptoms often become apparent at childhood or infancy. It is also called insulin-dependent diabetes mellitus (IDDM) because the insulin-dependent person must take daily injections of insulin to stay alive. Before the discovery of insulin in 1921, people only lived a few years after diagnosis.

The second form is called type 2, "adult onset diabetes," because it most often occurs about middle age. It is also called non-insulin-dependent diabetes mellitus (NIDDM), because type 2 is not necessarily a lack of insulin production, but rather the inability of the body to use it effectively.

We can do much with diet and exercise and other lifestyle modifications to alter the course of type 2. Some 90 percent of diabetics are type 2.

INSULIN AND ITS FUNCTIONS

Insulin functions in our body's sugar (carbohydrate) mechanisms. This hormone is made in scattered areas of the pancreas called Isles of Langerhans. These "islands" contain specialized cells called beta cells.

By the way, the "islands" were named in honor of the German pathologist Paul Langerhans, who first described them in 1869. He had no idea what function they performed. It wasn't until the 1920s that we discovered insulin.

There are many forms of sugar in our diet (sucrose, lactose, etc.), but before the body can use them, they must all be converted into glucose.

Once in the blood, the glucose must then enter individual cells where it is used for energy to run the cellular machinery. The hormone insulin from the pancreas is essential for glucose to get into the cell. Insulin is the only hormone in the body with this function.

There are two exceptions to the rule that insulin must be active to get glucose into the cell. This first has to do with the cells of the brain, where glucose can enter without insulin. The second exception is exercise, where the muscle cells can remove glucose from the blood without insulin (refer to page 46).

When it is working normally, the pancreas responds to every minute fluctuation in blood sugar. If blood sugar goes up, insulin is released; as blood sugar drops, insulin release is stopped. The system is much like a thermostat on your furnace. The thermostat turns the furnace off and on to maintain a constant temperature in your house.

Here is how the whole system works. When the blood sugar rises after we eat a meal, a signal goes to the pancreas to release insulin. Insulin (a storage hormone) moves the glucose from the blood into the cells for energy production. As the blood sugar drops, insulin shuts off until needed again.

Let's further simplify this mechanism to lay some groundwork we will use as we move along. Imagine that each of your cells has a door that must be opened to let glucose in. All doors have a doorknob. This is the insulin receptor. Think of insulin as the door opener for glucose to get into the cell.

So, you see, there can be two "blocks" to getting glucose inside the cell.

First, insulin (the door opener) can be absent or inefficient. Second, we can have a missing doorknob (the insulin receptor) or a doorknob that cannot be easily used for one reason or another.

WHAT HAPPENS IF THERE IS NO INSULIN?

As the blood sugar level rises rapidly, this results in the four classic symptoms of type 1 diabetes.

- **Frequent urination (Polyuria)**
  This happens because the kidneys are stimulated by the high glucose level to excrete a large volume of glucose-loaded urine to try to get the levels down. At normal levels of glucose,

the kidneys conserve glucose, so none is in the urine.

- **Excessive thirst (Polydipsia)**
  With all this urination going on, the individual becomes very thirsty and drinks large amount of fluids to replace the water loss.

- **Weight loss occurs**
  The cells cannot get food, so they begin to starve. This results in weight loss.

- **The cells send out "I'm starving" messages and your appetite increases**
  Despite excessive food intake, the weight loss continues because the cells cannot utilize the food you ingest.

If the situation is allowed to progress, the whole metabolism is totally thrown off and the blood becomes more acidic. This is called diabetic ketoacidosis. There is now great danger that the patient could go into a diabetic coma and die.

Those with type 1 diabetes nearly always need insulin injections, but the amount of insulin can usually be reduced by following the advice given in this chapter.

A CLOSE LOOK AT TYPE 1

The beta cells in the Isles of Langerhans that produce insulin are badly damaged or destroyed. They can no longer produce adequate insulin to control the blood sugar. The exact cause is not known, but it seems to be an interaction of four factors.

There is an inherited tendency towards type 1. Twin studies are most often used to determine whether a situation is inherited because their genetic makeup are identical. Several studies concerning identical twins have been done with type 1 diabetes in which one of the pair developed diabetes. The chance of the second twin developing the disease varies from 30 to 50 percent.

What this means is type 1 is not an absolutely inherited condition, but there is some genetic predisposition that increases a person's risk of the disease. To add to the mystery, severe type 1 can develop in people with no family history of any form of diabetes.

ATTACK ON THE "ISLAND"

Acute damage to beta cells can be caused by a variety of factors. Some viral diseases are definitely implicated. Diseases like flu, mumps, chickenpox and measles are all associated with the development of type 1. In one report, a young boy developed severe type 1 following a case of the flu. The virus that caused the boy's flu was isolated and injected into an experimental animal. The virus attacked and destroyed the beta cells, and the animal developed diabetes. Either there is something genetic that attracts these virus particles to the beta cells, or the immune system could be malfunctioning in some way.

There are also reports of environmental chemical compounds such as pesticides being a factor in the cause of type 1. Furthermore, some type 1 diabetics report an extremely stressful event occurring six to eight months before the onset of their diabetes. It is possible that stress, mild viral attacks and environmental chemicals combined with a genetically susceptible person are all involved in causing the disease.

The body's immune system cells produce antibodies (think of them as "bug spray") to kill an invading virus, bacteria or other foreign invaders. For some reason, these antibodies produced in response to one of the invaders above may attack the beta cells along with the invader. They treat the beta cells as though they were invaders. At least 32 percent of type 1 diabetics have antibodies that attack their own beta cells.

TYPE 2

Non-insulin-dependent diabetes mellitus (NIDDM) is by far the most common form of diabetes. It differs so much from type 1 that it almost seems to be an entirely different disease.

Quite often, type 2 has none of the classic symptoms of type 1 such as frequent urination, thirst, etc. As a matter of fact, it is most often discovered during a routine laboratory test of blood or urine.

The typical patient is overweight, middle-aged and inactive. There is a more solid genetic connection with type 2. In about 85 percent of cases, a parent or close relative has (or had) diabetes. So, if diabetes runs in your family, it is best to take precautions for prevention now.

The usual treatment consists of weight loss, diet modification, an exercise program, and sometimes an oral anti-diabetes medication.

In type 2, there is generally no problem with insulin production (the cell door opener). The problem is with the cell's insulin receptor (the door knob).

No matter how many door openers you have (insulin), if the door knob (insulin receptor) is not there, or is not functional, you cannot get the cell door to open to admit glucose and other nourishment for the cell. Fat is definitely involved.

To give a simple analogy for a complex situation, it's like fat makes the doorknob too slippery for the insulin to get a grip and open the door. This lack of insulin sensitivity is further illustrated by the fact that type 2 diabetics given insulin injections are often incapable of responding to the insulin. By just losing a few pounds, many type 2 diabetics can control their problem.

GESTATIONAL DIABETES

This occurs during pregnancy when hormonal changes accompanying pregnancy increase the body's resistance to insulin.

Women who are overweight and older are more prone to this type of diabetes. While it usually disappears after pregnancy, more than half of these women will develop type 2 diabetes later in life.

Women with this problem can also be prone to develop urinary tract infections and pre-eclampsia (pregnancy-induced hypertension), a condition unique to pregnancy.

A regular gentle exercise regime during pregnancy will help to lower blood glucose level.

The Dangers of Uncontrolled Sugar

Insulin does not cure diabetes. Insulin keeps you alive. Diabetics no longer die from elevated blood sugar levels. Instead, they have to contend with the long-term complications of the condition. To some degree or another, nearly all diabetics eventually have problems due to complications of the disease. Since one or more of these problems seem to be ubiquitous with diabetics, my goal is to help prevent the onset of these complications for as long as possible. This will help you with longevity, but perhaps even more importantly, greatly improve the quality of your life.

Over time, elevated blood sugar levels will lead to the following complications:

- Heart attack (atherosclerosis)
- Eye problem (retinopathy)
- Neurologic problems (neuropathy)
- High blood pressure
- Renal problems (kidney failure)
- Infections

Heart Attack
Continuous high sugar level over time will damage the blood vessels through the build up of atherosclerotic plaque, causing the narrowing of the arteries leading to the heart. Diabetics are especially prone to atherosclerosis. It is the cause of death of about 46 percent of the general population, but 75 percent of the diabetic population. Diabetics are also twice as likely to have strokes as the general population.

Diabetics have a predisposition towards abnormally high levels of fats circulating in the blood. This means high cholesterol and high triglycerides. A non-diabetic should take precautions against heart disease but a diabetic needs to do everything possible to protect the blood vessels from damage.

Diabetic Retinopathy

The small vessels leading to the retina can become damaged, causing loss of vision or blindness (diabetic retinopathy). Nine out of 10 diabetics within 20 years will show damage to their retina. This is the lining at the back of the eye where light is received and then sent to the brain.

There are two types of diabetic retinopathy. The first is known as simple retinopathy or background retinopathy. The blood vessels in this area narrow, thus cutting down the oxygen supply to the eyes. Later, they can weaken and small hemorrhages could occur.

With background retinopathy, control of sugar levels and especially control of blood pressure is important. High blood pressure, even without diabetes, can cause retinopathy. Also, controlling the risk factors for heart disease is excellent protection. Hard work in these areas should delay the onset of background retinopathy, but does not usually reverse it.

About one in five progress to the second form: proliferative retinopathy. It is characterized by the growth of new blood vessels within the retina and scarring. It works like this: Capillaries along the inner surface of the retina start multiplying or proliferating, probably as a response to decreased oxygen supply to the eye. These new blood vessels try to bring more oxygen into the area, but they are very fragile vessels; they can break and bleed into various parts of the eye. Blurred vision can result and scarring can cause a detached retina. This is obviously a much more serious problem than background retinopathy and needs attention immediately.

Diabetic Neuropathy

Nerve functions are also affected. Some of the symptoms are tingling, pins and needles sensation, burning, itching, numbness and, sometimes, severe pain. Most of the time it is not constant, but it comes and goes. Neuropathy most often affects the legs and feet. Narrowing of the medium-sized arteries to the legs and feet, penis and skin can lead to:

- Gangrene. Foot ulcers heal so poorly that part of the leg may have to be amputated.
- Impotence in men (poor supply of blood to the penis).
- Poor healing of any wound.

High Blood Pressure
The high blood pressure seems to go along with the narrowing of the diameter of the blood vessels. Many cases of high blood pressure are still a mystery to the medical profession.

Renal Problems
The younger the age of the onset, the longer the duration of diabetes, and the less you control your sugar, the more likely you are to have diabetic kidney problems. Almost all insulin-dependent diabetics have some kidney damage, but for most, it does not cause symptoms or problems. About 35 percent develop kidney problems, usually around 15 to 20 years after diagnosis. Kidney failure accounts for 48 percent of all deaths in diabetics who acquire the disease before age 20.

I am a strong believer in prevention. So, if you are diabetic and all of your kidney studies are presently normal, I would still begin a program of prevention. This means to be extremely careful in controlling your blood sugar. It also means to be selective in your protein consumption.

Infections
Diabetics are more prone to infections than non-diabetics. This means a diabetic must keep his or her immune system in optimal condition. I recommend you read my book on the *Immune System*.

Dietary Control – Glycemic Index and Glycemic Load

Our dietary strategy is to use food to control blood glucose level to as near normal as possible. This will help prevent or slow the progress of many long-term complications associated with diabetes such as blindness, heart disease, kidney failure and gangrene leading to amputation.

THE GLYCEMIC INDEX

The best diet for a person with diabetes is to use diet therapy to help maintain a blood sugar level to as near normal as possible. The diet should include:

- Low intake of saturated fat, trans fat, cholesterol, salt and sugar
- Moderate consumption of alcohol
- Plenty of fresh, colorful vegetables and fruits rich in nutrients, antioxidants and phytochemicals
- Moderate amounts of lean meat

The real problem is carbohydrate; it is the only part of food that has a direct impact on sugar levels in the blood compared to fats and protein. As we cannot predict how a carbohydrate behaves in the body just by looking at the sugar or starch content, researchers developed an index called the Glycemic Index (GI), which ranks carbohydrate food by how fast 50 grams of a carbohydrate of a particular food is converted into glucose and enters the bloodstream.

Pure glucose or white bread has a ranking of 100 on the GI and all other carbohydrates are ranked in relation to glucose. High GI foods cause blood glucose to rise quickly, resulting in higher levels of insulin in the blood, while low GI foods cause a steady rise in blood glucose. Generally, foods that undergo the least processing have low GI.

However, a food is not good or bad solely because of its GI values. A high GI food may significantly increase the risk of heart disease besides diabetes and obesity but when you are choosing foods, GI isn't the only thing to consider. You should also consider the amount of calories, the type of fat, fiber, salt, vitamin and mineral content.

However, knowing the GI of a food may be helpful for a diabetic when it comes to timing meals and medication to maintain blood glucose level to as near normal as possible to avoid diabetic complications.

The glycemic effect of foods can be lowered by:

- Not over-consuming carbohydrates at any one time of the day

- Eating starchy carbohydrate foods in combination with lean protein, fiber and fats which will slow down absorption of sugar into the blood

- Eating vegetable and grains in whole form whenever possible – "nature-made" carbohydrates usually have low GI compared to "man-made" carbohydrates

- Distributing intake of carbohydrates throughout the day: three big meals and two snacks in between to keep blood glucose level to as near normal as possible – eating like a deer (grazing throughout the day) is better than eating like a bear (a few big meals)

- Eating dried beans and peas to lower the glycemic effect of other foods

GLYCEMIC INDEX OF CARBOHYDRATE FOODS

Michael Mason in his book, *The Insulin Threat: Carbohydrates and Your Heart* lists some general categories of the glycemic index of foods, with recommendation for people with diabetes or insulin resistance:

High GI Foods
- Grains and starches, pasta, bread, bagel, cereals, potatoes and all processed food in general
- Candies, honey and table sugar
- Grain based snacks – corn chips, cookies, etc.
- Prepared cereals – cornflakes, muesli and instant cereals
- Certain fruits – bananas, raisins and most fruit juice
- Starchy vegetables, potatoes and corn

Moderate GI Foods
- Canned legumes and frozen peas
- Sweet potatoes and yams
- Whole grain cereals

Low GI Foods
- Certain fruits – cherries, grapes, grapefruit, peaches, plums, apples, pears and oranges
- Legumes – freshly cooked black-eyed beans, chickpeas, kidney beans, lentils and soy beans
- Non-starchy vegetables – asparagus, bok choy, broccoli, cabbage, celery, lettuce, mushrooms, spinach, sweet potato, tomatoes and green pepper

According to Dr. Jennie Miller, author of *The Glucose Revolution Power Guide to Diabetes*: "Low GI foods have values over 55 or below, intermediate GI values at between 55 and 70, and high GI values more than 70."

GLYCEMIC LOAD (GL)

We learnt earlier that GI is concerned about how rapidly 50 grams of a particular carbohydrate turn into glucose and spike insulin levels in the body, but it does not indicate the amount of carbohydrate in the food. The amount of carbohydrates consumed also affects blood glucose levels and insulin responses. For example, carrots have a high glycemic index of 92 that is almost the same as sugar but a Glycemic Load (GL) of 5. You would have to eat boxes and boxes of them to have any pronounced effect on blood sugar. This is because the amount of carbohydrates in a carrot is very small. Besides, it is rich in nutrients.

Or take watermelon as another example. A slice of watermelon, a sweet tasting fruit, has a high GI of 72 but with a GL of 4. This is because a watermelon is made up mostly of water but has only a small amount of carbohydrates per serving. While the GI value is a helpful gauge, it doesn't always reveal the whole story when choosing which carbohydrate to eat. This is where the GL comes in. It is an offshoot of the glycemic index popularized by Harvard nutritionist Walter Willett.

Glycemic load is a rating based on the GI and amount of carbohydrate eaten. It can be used to describe the effects of one food; a meal; a whole day's eating; or eating over many days. In many recent studies, the glycemic load of a person's overall diet is more significant than the glycemic index of individual foods.

The glycemic load of a food is calculated by multiplying the glycemic index by the actual number of grams of carbohydrate eaten in a meal and dividing the total by 100. As an example, take watermelon with a high glycemic index of 72. A serving of 120 grams contains 6 grams of available carbohydrates, so its glycemic load is calculated as: 72 (GI) x 6 /100 = 4.32, rounded to 4.

Foods high in GL have been associated with an increased risk of developing type 2 diabetes. The Nurses' Health Study showed that women with the highest dietary glycemic loads were 37 percent more likely to develop type 2 over the next six years than women with the lowest dietary glycemic loads (*JAMA*. 1997; 277(6):472-477).

GI and GL values for selected foods

See the table below for the glycemic index and glycemic load values of selected foods. A GL of a food is considered low if its value is 10 or less; a medium from 11-19; and high if it is 20 or more.

Glycemic Index and Glycemic Load Values for Selected Foods (Relative to Glucose)

Food	Glycemic Index (Glucose=100)	Serving size	Carbohydrates per serving (g)	Glycemic Load per serving
Dates, dried	103	2 oz	40	42
Cornflakes	81	1 cup	26	21
Jelly beans	78	1 oz	28	22
Puffed rice cakes	78	3 cakes	21	17
Russet potato (baked)	76	1 medium	30	23
Doughnut	76	1 medium	23	17
Soda crackers	74	4 crackers	17	12
White bread	73	1 large slice	14	10
Table sugar (sucrose)	68	2 tsp	10	7
Pancake	67	6" diameter	58	39
White rice (boiled)	64	1 cup	36	23
Brown rice (boiled)	55	1 cup	33	18
Spaghetti, white; boiled 10-15 min	44	1 cup	40	18
Spaghetti, white; boiled 5 min	38	1 cup	40	15
Spaghetti, whole wheat; boiled	37	1 cup	37	14
Rye, pumpernickel bread	41	1 large slice	12	5
Oranges, raw	42	1 medium	11	5
Pears, raw	38	1 medium	11	4
Apples, raw	38	1 medium	15	6
All-Bran™ cereal	38	1 cup	23	9
Skim milk	32	8 fl oz	13	4
Lentils, dried; boiled	29	1 cup	18	5
Kidney beans, dried; boiled	28	1 cup	25	7
Pearled barley; boiled	25	1 cup	42	11
Cashew nuts	22	1 oz	9	2
Peanuts	14	1 oz	6	1

Source: Jane Higdon, Ph.D. Linus Pauling Institute, Oregon State University.

BOTTOM LINE

The GI and GL are useful for people with normal glucose metabolism but it is more important to people with diabetes and pre-diabetes. When preparing meals or eating out, use the GI and GL of a carbohydrate as a guide with the objective of keeping your blood glucose stable, to help control appetite, improve weight loss, lower LDL cholesterol, raise HDL cholesterol and improve insulin resistance.

This action helps reduce your risk of heart disease and pre-diabetes, and prevent diabetes from taking hold of your body. "Nature-made" carbohydrates containing soluble and insoluble fibers are better than "man-made" carbohydrates which undergo refining or are highly processed.

Products made from grains (corn) and tubers (potatoes), which grow above the ground, are mostly high in GI and GL. Foods with large particle sizes, high fiber content and high acidity have lower GI compared to processed food with little fiber and small particle sizes. Raw foods have a lower GI than cooked food.

Overall, the theory of "glycemic index" and "glycemic load" encourages you to reduce your intake of refined carbohydrates and increase your diet with foods high in antioxidants such as carotenoids, lycopene, lutein, zeaxanthin and bioflavonoids, mainly from a variety of fresh vegetables and low sugar fruits.

When you are choosing foods, you should also consider the amount of calories, the amount and type of fat, fiber, salt, vitamin and mineral content besides the quality and quantity of a carbohydrate food.

LOW FAT AND LEAN PROTEIN

Monounsaturated fats (canola or olive oil) or polyunsaturated fats (sunflower, soy or corn oil) are acceptable as long as they do not contain trans fatty acids resulting from hydrogenation.

Keep away from fatty red meat, organ meat, processed foods with plenty of additives, coloring and preservatives, fried foods, fast food, foods rich in saturated fats and high cholesterol food.

Consume protein foods such as tofu, egg white, chicken without skin, fish rich in omega-3 fatty acid like salmon, cod, tuna and herring, lean meat, low-fat dairy products, turkey and a good vegetable protein drink.

Nutrients of Benefit

Besides diet, I want to focus in this chapter on how food supplements and herbs can help prevent or delay the onset of long-term diabetic complications.

THE FOUNDATION

Every endeavor needs a good foundation on which to build. The foundation for a diabetic supplement program is the multi-vitamin/mineral. We do not always eat as we should for one reason (excuse) or another, so the multi is insurance for those times. You are attempting to replace nutrients that may be short or missing in your diet; this is the logical place to begin.

FIBER

Soluble fiber helps prevent drastic shifts in blood sugar levels, making it an attractive weapon in the war against diabetes. Foods high in soluble fiber include fruits, vegetables, oats and dried beans.

Many studies show that increasing soluble fiber in the diet can lower total cholesterol. For most people, soluble fiber targets the "bad" LDL faction and leaves the "good" HDL alone. These fibers bind cholesterol in the intestine and prevent it from being reabsorbed. Cholesterol is simply excreted.

To help with the fiber problem, it is easier to add a good quality fiber supplement. This way, only one food is being added to the diet, and it is easier to work in without upsetting the body chemistry too much. It makes it easier to figure because you are adding a known and measured amount to each meal. Along with your supplement, slowly add in other dietary fiber sources, but monitor your sugar carefully as you do so.

For more details on fiber please read my book entitled *Why a fiber supplement?*

CHROMIUM

Chromium increases the power of insulin to process sugar. With adequate chromium in the blood, the level of insulin required in circulation is reduced.

This reduces your risk of developing atherosclerosis and long-term diabetic complications.

Chromium can help improve insulin resistance in diabetics. In one study, a daily consumption of 200 mcg of chromium improved insulin resistance in 62 percent of the women and 50 percent of men with type 2 diabetes, within 10 days.

The best supplemental forms are chromium polynicotinate and chromium picolinate. Chromium is safe when taken at a dosage of 50 to 200 mcg daily. No side effects have been noted.

If you are on insulin, take chromium under your doctor's supervision. He may need to adjust your insulin dosage as your blood sugar level drops.

EICOSAPENTAENOIC ACID (EPA)

Two essential fatty acids, EPA and DHA, have been shown to have a beneficial effect on the vascular system where diabetic problems are concerned. They are found in cold-water fish such as mackerel, haddock, sardines, anchovies, and some salmon and tuna. The American Heart Association has urged us to add these fish to our usual diets.

So far as the vascular system goes, diabetics tend to have the following problems:

- They run higher levels of blood lipids such as triglycerides and cholesterol.

- Their blood platelets, which are responsible for beginning a blood clot, tend to be more sticky and bond together easily, thus interfering with blood flow. This is called platelet aggregation.

- Their red blood cells can become somewhat inflexible, making it hard for these cells to enter very small capillaries. This reduces the oxygen supply to the tissues.

- Due to structural changes, their small blood vessels become constricted.

- They also tend to have higher blood pressure.

EPA lowers triglycerides. Low triglycerides are associated with high HDL levels, so as triglycerides go down, HDL generally goes up. EPA changes the configuration of some chemical messengers in the body called prostaglandins. As a result, the blood platelets are less sticky and platelet aggregation is reduced. EPA helps the red blood cells to be more flexible and fit through small capillaries better. Additionally, the blood flows more smoothly, blood vessels are slightly dilated, and in some studies EPA has lowered high blood pressure.

EPA sounds like a diabetic's dream, but you will hear of a couple of studies that report the following:

"LDL cholesterol levels were mildly elevated" and "Fasting glucose levels were elevated." But in light of all of the benefits for a diabetic's vascular system, I would tend to go along with another report that says: "The mild LDL increase is not significant compared with the other anti-atherosclerotic effects of omega-3 fatty acids, and the slight elevation of fasting glucose can be controlled."

Since EPA has an effect on blood clotting and blood flow

similar to that of aspirin, it should be of help in early background retinopathy. The increased flow and slowing of platelet clumping should allow more oxygen to get to the eye.

The only caution is, if you have a retinopathy that has advanced to the stage of leaking capillaries, you should avoid aspirin and high levels of EPA.

GAMMA LINOLENIC ACID (GLA)

Diabetic neuropathy is one of the most common of all diabetic complications. It seems to be the result of the effect of diabetes on both blood vessels and nerves. It can also manifest itself through a loss of tendon reflexes and muscle strength. Various studies on GLA indicate it can have some very positive effects on diabetic neuropathy by affecting the nerves and helping the blood supply.

Is GLA lacking? It is well accepted that the conversion process of dietary linolenic acid (the main unsaturated fat from vegetables) to GLA is inadequate in diabetic patients. A lack of GLA causes problems with the sheath covering the nerves (myelin sheath) and reduces blood flow. Therefore, adding the essential fatty acid GLA should have important implications in the approach to prevention and treatment of diabetic neuropathy. The main sources of GLA are evening primrose oil and borage oil seed.

EXTREMELY VITAL VITAMIN E

Dr. Wilfrid Shute and his brother Dr. Evan Shute worked with over 35,000 patients at the Shute Clinic in London, Ontario. They were among the first to begin reporting the near miraculous effectiveness of vitamin E in the body. During their years of study they reported the following benefits of vitamin E which concern diabetics:

• Helps dissolve fresh clots in veins

- Reduces the oxygen requirements of tissues and cells
- Helps form new skin (in healing burns and ulcers)
- Helps ulcers that seem unlikely to heal
- Increases the blood supply to tissues and thus reduces diabetic gangrene and amputations
- Reduces the need for insulin in 30 percent of diabetics on vitamin E
- Prevents the platelets from clumping together to form dangerous pre-clots

Vitamin E has also been reported to help in some forms of neuropathy. It relieves "restless feet" syndrome and has been most effective in various neuropathies, especially the tingling feeling in feet and legs.

Due to its effect in widening some blood vessels, it should be of benefit in background retinopathy.

AM I EXCITED?

Now do you see why I am so excited about vitamin E? This is simply an amazing nutrient for diabetics. How much is too much? Vitamin E is extremely safe. Dr. Lawrence Machlin and his colleagues at the Cornell Medical School summarized the vitamin E safety issue clearly. In studies where people took from 600 to 3,200 IU of vitamin E a day, no negative side effects were reported. There is only one caution. Vitamin E interacts with vitamin K. If you are deficient in vitamin K or are on medication to prevent blood clotting, you should take high levels of vitamin E only under medical guidance.

Personally, I take 800 IU a day. I feel comfortable with that number for the present time. Be sure you take a natural vitamin E. It will be labeled d-alpha tocopherol. The label should also state that it contains the entire spectrum of vitamin E as it exists in nature. The natural form has been proven to work better in the body.

OH SAY CAN YOU "C"

Reams of evidence have been appearing in research literature indicating that vitamin C ingested in amounts well above the DV will offer enhanced health benefits and possible protection against some diseases.

Vitamin C is extremely important for us because it is involved in so many areas of health. When stress hits, vitamin C is used up at a fantastic rate. It is involved in the production of several adrenal hormones. Vitamin C protects us against a number of airborne pollutants. As it protects, it is used up, so we need a continuous re-supply. It will reduce the duration of a cold and at the same time reduce its unpleasant symptoms.

Vitamin C is essential in the healing of wounds, and if you bruise easily, you may be low in vitamin C. This remarkable vitamin also stimulates your immune system to be more aggressive, which is very important to diabetics because of their risk of catching an infection.

Vitamin C may have a very important role in the prevention of heart disease by preventing the oxidation of LDL cholesterol into an even more deadly form. This remarkable vitamin protects and preserves vitamin E. This nutrient can strengthen capillaries and other blood vessels, making them less likely to leak blood into the tissues. This is extremely vital in some forms of retinopathy.

B COMPLEX

The B complex is another important set of vitamins for the diabetic. The whole complex is intimately involved in sugar metabolism and energy release.

In neuropathy (especially pain or burning symptoms) about 80 percent experience some improvement with the B complex. Many report complete relief.

Some members of the B complex have been reported to increase glucose utilization in diabetics. This would be especially helpful for type 2 diabetics. The complex has also helped those with leg ulcers. They help cure the ulcer and also prevent its recurrence. In fact, diabetics may have much higher requirement for B6 than the normal population. This vitamin is necessary for the normal metabolism of an amino acid called tryptophan.

Abnormal metabolism of this amino acid causes a form of diabetes. When B6 is supplemented, diabetes in some cases improves significantly. Also, B6 supplementation may reverse some forms of diabetes that are associated with pregnancy.

ZINC

Zinc is a most valuable mineral to diabetics. Insulin contains an amazing amount of zinc. Diabetics tend to have higher zinc requirements. There seem to be several reasons for this. One, because so much is lost in the urine, diabetics need more replacements. Second, a diabetic's pancreas contains only about half the amount of stored zinc in a normal pancreas. This means a diabetic has a lower storage capacity than normal.

The skin contains about 20 percent of the body's total zinc. It is there for a good reason. Zinc aids in the process of healing wounds. Diabetics tend to be plagued with skin ulcers, and optimal zinc is essential for their healing and to prevent their recurrence.

Zinc can also stimulate the immune system. Several studies have shown that the immune systems in older people become much more active when they consume supplemental zinc. A diabetic needs an immune system that is at high levels of efficiency all the time.

CALCIUM AND MAGNESIUM

Biochemically, magnesium has a fundamental role in carbohydrate metabolism, and a very specific role in the efficient action of insulin.

A low level of magnesium can certainly contribute to poor control of the diabetic condition.

The diabetic condition itself may cause a reduction in magnesium levels. Also, elevated sugar levels cause an increase in urination, which can wash out magnesium. Whatever the multifaceted reasons, the diabetic condition predisposes the patient to a magnesium deficiency.

We know low levels of magnesium are associated with heart disease. But this is even more serious for diabetics due to their propensity for heart disease.

ALPHA LIPOIC ACID

Five years ago, hardly anybody heard of alpha lipoic acid. Today, we know that like coenzyme Q10, alpha lipoic acid is involved in the conversion of carbohydrates and fats into energy. Like coenzyme Q10, vitamins A, C, and E, alpha lipoic acid is an antioxidant.

Perhaps the most widely noted clinical application of alpha lipoic acid is the treatment of diabetes and its complications. Alpha lipoic acid is critical for diabetics because it increases the uptake and utilization of glucose and improves blood sugar control in both type 1 and type 2 diabetes. Glycation – the process by which glucose combines with proteins – is a major cause of tissue destruction in diabetes, resulting in neuropathy, kidney damage and retinal injury that can lead to blindness. Alpha lipoic acid blocks these conditions, while protecting and healing injuries to the eyes, kidneys and nerves.

Diabetics generally have low levels of alpha lipoic acid and it is important for them to receive it as a supplement. To ensure adequate amounts of alpha lipoic acid, a typical dose is 100 mg a day. For individuals with complications, the dose may need to be increased up to 300 mg to 600 mg a day.

Herbal Stars

Here are six star herbs that can help you control your sugar levels or in your management of diabetic complications.

GARLIC

There are numerous scientific research indicating that garlic can play a role in the prevention and management of diabetic complications. There is still some debate as to how it works. One theory is that it increases the efficiency of insulin output. Another is that it stimulates the liver to be more effective in removing sugar from the blood.

It is probably more effective in type 2 diabetes than type 1. Garlic can dramatically lower the blood level of both cholesterol and triglycerides. It has a tendency to thin the blood and is an immune system enhancer. If I had diabetes, I would certainly give it a try.

GINKGO BILOBA

Usually in our thirties, the brain's ability to process information begins to slow down. Here is the reason. Just as plaque deposits in the arteries of the heart, it also deposits in the blood vessels of the brain. This lack of blood supply to the brain nerve cells results in cerebral insufficiency.

Ginkgo can help improve blood flow through arteries, veins and capillaries. It can be of great help in preventing or reversing cerebral insufficiency. Since diabetics tend to have more vessel blockage than those without diabetes, I strongly urge you to use this herb.

In other studies, ginkgo improved eye function in diabetic patients with early stage retinopathy after six months of supplementation as compared to placebo treated controls (*Journal French Ophthalmol* 1988: 11 (10): 71-4).

84

Recommended dosage is 120 mg daily, divided into three doses of 40 mg pills.

BILBERRY

Bilberry contains a powerful antioxidant, anthocyanosides, that has been used in traditional herbal medicine to treat glaucoma, cataracts, macular degeneration and diabetic retinopathy. In Europe, bilberry is used frequently for both the treatment and prevention of diabetic retinopathy.

Clinical studies support the fact that bilberry has the ability to lower blood sugar, even when blood sugar level is abnormally high (*Quarterly Journal Crude Drug Res*, 1979, 17: 139-196).

Look for a standardized extract with not less than 25 percent content of anthocyanosides. The standard dosage is 120 to 240 mg twice daily.

FENUGREEK

Results of both animal and human studies favor the use of fenugreek seeds (an Indian spice plant) to lower blood sugar levels in type 2 diabetes. One study on diabetes with coronary artery disease found both blood glucose and lipids lowered in type 2 diabetes after three months of consuming 2.5 grams of fenugreek seeds (*Prostaglandins, Leukotrines and Essential Fatty Acids,* 1997).

Yet in another study, diabetics given 25 grams divided equally into two meals for 24 weeks observed improvement in fasting blood glucose, insulin level and improved glucose tolerance. The abundant fiber and gum content of the seeds appears to be the major contributor to its glucose lowering effects (*European Journal of Clinical Nutrition,* 1998), thus slowing glucose's rate of entry into the bloodstream.

Because of the bitterness of fenugreek seeds, it is advisable to take them in capsule form. Avoid this herb during pregnancy.

GYMNEMA SYLVESTRE

This is a traditional Ayurvedic herb, found in the tropical forests of India and has long been used as a treatment for diabetes. Gymnemic acid is claimed to be the active ingredient, a chemically complex mixture of saponins.

In one important study, 400 mg of gymnema sylvestre given to 22 type 2 diabetics for 20 months, reported lower blood sugar and glycosylated hemoglobin. Many lowered their intake of their diabetic medication and five discontinued their medication altogether and remained on gymnema extract to control their blood sugar level (*Journal Ethnopharmacol* 1990 Oct; 30 (3): 295-300).

Look for a standardized extract to contain 24 percent gymnemic acid. It is usually taken at a dosage of 400-600 mg daily.

BITTER MELON (Momordica charantia)

Bitter melon, also known as balsam pear, is a tropical vegetable used extensively in folk medicine as a remedy for diabetes. In both experimental and clinical studies, the blood sugar lowering action of the fresh juice or extract of the unripe fruit has been established clearly. Research suggests that bitter melon helps increase the number of beta cells in the pancreas, thereby improving the body's ability to produce insulin.

Excessively high doses of bitter melon juice can cause abdominal pain and diarrhea. Anyone with hypoglycemia should not take bitter melon. Diabetics taking oral medication for diabetes or insulin should take bitter melon with caution.

Go for a Healthy Lifestyle

Because there is no cure for diabetes, it's important that you make changes in your lifestyle to help you live comfortably with the disease and avoid serious long-term diabetic complications. Here are some suggested lifestyle guidelines that can help you manage your diabetes for a lifetime of good health:

- Plan your meal. Remember you should use diet as the first line of defense against the risk of developing diabetes. Taking your meals on a regular timetable will keep your sugar level steady. Skipping meals can cause your blood sugar level to drop too much (hypoglycemia), while overeating will cause your sugar level to rise too high (hyperglycemia).

- Exercise can help keep your sugar under control and actually lower your insulin requirements. It has been called the "invisible insulin." The more exercise you get (if you are in good health), the less insulin you are likely to require and the more stable your diabetes will be. Exercise helps in a number of areas that are of vital concern to diabetics. Individuals with this disease are very prone to heart disease. Further, exercise lowers the level of glucose circulating in the blood. It is especially beneficial for type 2 diabetics.

  Exercise not only increases the number of insulin receptors on the cells, it also increases the insulin sensitivity of these receptors. In one study at Yale University Medical Center, a 50 percent increase in insulin receptors and a 30 percent increase in insulin sensitivity were demonstrated after a six-week program of daily exercise. Always consult with your physician before you begin an exercise program. For many, insulin requirements will change.

- Obesity is definitely associated with reduced insulin sensitivity. Fat in the body has a direct effect on the insulin receptors; many people can control type 2 by just losing some fat pounds.

  Your ideal weight is to keep your Body Mass Index (a simple index of weight-to-height ratio) between 20 and 25. If your BMI is above 26, you are more prone to develop weight-related diseases such as heart disease and diabetes, and these sharply rise with BMIs over 30. The BMI is calculated as:

$$\frac{\underline{Weight}}{Height \times Height}$$

- Another way to determine whether you are at a healthy weight is to measure your waist circumference. You put yourself at great risk of diabetes if your measurement exceeds 40 inches, if you are a man; and, 35 inches if you are a woman, especially if your BMI is 25-35.

- Monitor your blood glucose regularly to take better care of your diabetes. You can measure your sugar level with the help of a test strip or a glucose meter. They are easily available in most pharmacies.

- Practice good foot and skin care. Take special care of your feet.

- Do not smoke anything. Diabetics have a much greater tendency towards heart and other vascular disease. Smoking is well known to make these problems much worse. Smoking constricts the blood vessels in the heart, as well as the smaller vessels in the legs and feet. This reduces circulation and causes tissues to heal more slowly.

  Diabetics are susceptible to foot and leg ulcers, and smoking compounds the problem. Diabetics tend to have less oxygen in their tissues than other people. Smoking raises the level of carbon monoxide in the blood, thus adding to the oxygen deficit.

- Try to manage stress as best as you can. Any sort of practice that will lower your stress such as bio-feedback, meditation, hypnotherapy or other relaxation techniques may help lessen your insulin requirement.

- Always wear a medic alert or tag, or carry your medical smart card with you, in case you have a hypoglycemic attack.

- Drink at least eight glasses of purified water everyday. Water is the precious transport fluid that helps carry waste and nutrients. As the quality of our water has become questionable, I suggest a good quality water purifier which carries the National Sanitation Foundation (NSF) seal. The seal guarantees quality.

- Follow your medication schedule as prescribed by your doctor.

- Go for regular checkups.

- Get regular eye examinations.

Just working on these guidelines can go a long way in controlling some forms of diabetes and, most importantly, limit the complications associated with diabetes.

Diagnosis and Treatment of Diabetes

If you are experiencing symptoms of diabetes, there are several different blood tests available to determine whether you have diabetes. These tests are either before a meal or after taking a meal or a pre-measured glucose drink. Glucose tests are used to determine whether or not your blood glucose level is within the normal range. They are also used to screen for, diagnose and monitor patients with diabetes and pre-diabetes. These tests cannot determine whether you have type 1 or type 2 diabetes.

Healthy people without diabetes are recommended to test for diabetes before 45 and again after three years. Diabetes begins its painless destruction at lower sugar levels than previously thought. High blood sugar produces no symptoms, and many adults have diabetes for seven years or more before it is diagnosed. By that time, irreversible damage to the circulatory system and organs may have already occurred.

FASTING BLOOD GLUCOSE (BLOOD SUGAR) LEVEL

This is the standard test for diabetes. You are required to fast for 12 hours the night before. Your doctor will take a sample of your blood sugar to test your blood glucose level. See Table 1 on page 40 for guidelines.

ORAL GLUCOSE TOLERANCE TEST (OGTT)

The objective of this test is to find out how your body can handle excess sugar after drinking a high dose of a glucose drink.

Like the fasting glucose test, you do a 12-hour fast the night before. But this time, after your blood sample has been taken, you are given a glucose drink with 200-300 ml of water. For the next two hours, your blood sample will be taken by your doctor half hourly. Your results will be plotted on a glucose tolerance graph. Deviations from the normal can then be determined.

To test for the presence of diabetes, different dosages of a glucose drink will be given. In the case of men and non-pregnant women, a 75-gram glucose drink is used; a 100-gram drink is used for pregnant women to test for gestational diabetes. See Table 2 on page 40 and Table 3 below for guidelines.

**Table 3: Guideline of OGTT for pregnant women
after a 100-gram glucose drink to test for gestational diabetes**

When	Above-normal results for OGTT (mg/dL)
Fasting	Above 95 gestational diabetes
At 1 hour	Above 180 gestational diabetes
At 2 hours	Above 155 gestational diabetes
At 3 hours	Above 140 gestational diabetes

RANDOM BLOOD GLUCOSE TEST

A random plasma glucose test is just that: random at the laboratory. It can be done at any time. You don't have to fast to have this test.

Health professionals will sometimes use a random blood glucose test when they notice signs of diabetes during an appointment. Any abnormal test results should be followed up with either the fasting blood glucose test or the glucose tolerance test.

Blood samples are taken shortly after eating or drinking. Several random measurements may be taken throughout the day. Random testing is useful because glucose levels in healthy people do not vary widely throughout the day.

Blood glucose levels that are higher than 200 mg/dL may indicate a problem. The test allows the diabetic to carefully monitor blood glucose levels to assure that they are within normal range.

Table 4: Random glucose test guideline

Reading (mg/dL)	Diagnosis
Below 140	Normal
From 140 to 200	Pre-diabetes
Above 200	Diabetes

HEMOGLOBIN A1c (HbA1c) TEST

If your sugar level stays too high, it may be advisable to go for a test called HbA1c at least once every three months until your sugar level improves. This can only be done in a laboratory.

Hemoglobin is a substance in all red blood cells that carry oxygen throughout the body. When the level of glucose is too high, the sugar binds with the hemoglobin and the glucose may stay attached until the cell dies, which takes about three months. Measuring your HbA1c level thus offers you a picture of your blood glucose levels over the last three months.

The ideal range for HbA1c is generally less than 7 percent. Sometimes, healthy habits such as dietary control, losing weight and exercising are not enough to keep your blood glucose level under control; in that case your doctor may have you take diabetic medications or insulin injections. See Table 5 for guidelines.

Table 5: HbA1c mean plasma glucose

Approximate *HbA1c* Mean Plasma Glucose

HbA1c percent	mg/dL	mmol/L	Interpretation
4	65	3.5	
5	100	5.5	Non-Diabetic Range
6	135	7.5	
7	170	9.5	American Diabetic Association Target
8	205	11.5	
9	240	13.5	
10	275	15.5	Above Target
11	310	17.5	
12	345	19.5	

MEDICATION

If lifestyle, diet and food supplementation are not enough, diabetics may require drug therapy. Most drugs available in the market work by releasing more insulin from the pancreas or decreasing glucose output through the liver. There are several other medications available to treat diabetes and are only available by prescription through your doctor.

You should consult your doctor before taking any medication for diabetes. Even when you are on a drug or insulin injection, you should still continue to lead a healthy lifestyle.

THERE IS NO MAGIC

To some degree, diabetes eventually affects all the organs and systems of the body. Many of the medical problems of diabetics are no different from those other people have, but they occur more often, earlier, and seem to progress more rapidly. Some seem to simply accelerate the natural aging process, especially in the large blood vessels. But others are quite specific to diabetes, particularly those in the smaller blood vessels and the nervous system.

We have no magic cure, but early careful attention to your diabetic condition can reap great rewards later down the road.

The advice given here is meant to be used in conjunction with the advice given to you by your doctor concerning your specific situation. Of course, there are no guarantees in diabetes or any other disease, but one guarantee always holds true. Poor nutrition will give you a poor response to your disease. Optimal nutrition and lifestyle will give you the best possible chance for a better result during the course of the disease.

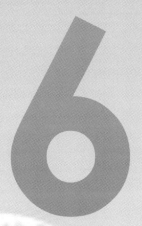

THE CHOLESTEROL CONNECTION

The Numbers Confusion

Are you confused by all of the lipid (blood fat) terms such as HDL, LDL, total cholesterol, saturated, monounsaturated, etc.? We are going to make all the healthy terms and numbers make sense, so that you will know their importance to you and your heart's health. Some people get so confused and frustrated that they throw up their hands in disgust and head for the local fast food (grease pit) establishment for a quick coronary "lube" job. Don't give up! Keep reading!

ANN'S STORY

"What are all of these numbers we are supposed to know?" Ann exclaimed to her friend while waving a sheet of paper containing her current blood lipids.

"My cholesterol is 210 mg/dL and my doctor says don't worry about it, but then I read in a magazine that 210 mg/dL is high," sighed Ann. "Also, what in the world are triglycerides, LDLs, HDLs and all of that other stuff?" Ann shook her head in worry. "I know I am supposed to increase fiber in my diet; I wonder if lettuce is high in fiber?" Ann gave an angry grimace, "I sometimes just feel like giving up; this is so confusing."

Ann is right; there is lot of confusion. The purpose of this chapter is to give some clear, concise and workable information. I will explain the "blood lipid profile" values, and give you reasonable ways to decrease your chances of a heart attack.

Most people can cut their risk of heart attack by 50 percent if they are willing to make a few simple changes in their lifestyles. The evidence is overwhelming!

By the way, Ann, who has the cholesterol reading of 210 mg/dL, is 70 years old, walks three miles a day, has never smoked, is at her exact weight and is taking two courses at a local university.

She should probably be more worried about her college grades than her cholesterol at 210 mg/dL.

A NOTE ON NUMBERS

In the United States, cholesterol is measured in milligrams per deciliter (mg/dL). In some countries, it is measured in millimoles per liter (mmol/L). The conversion formulas are:

Cholesterol Number Conversion
mg/dL of cholesterol x 0.02586 = mmol/L
mmol/L of cholesterol x 38.67   = mg/dL

Triglyceride Number Conversion
mg/dL of triglyceride x 0.01129 = mmol/L
mmol/L of triglyceride x 88.496 = mg/dL

HERE IS THE GOOD NEWS

Why do I say many can reduce their chances of dying from a heart attack by as much as 50 percent? Solid research reports that for each one percent reduction in blood cholesterol, you decrease your chances of a heart attack by an amazing two percent! Some studies are even indicating the reduction may approach three percent.

Let's pick a number that most people can easily achieve in four to six weeks on the plan we are going to suggest. Lower your cholesterol by only 10 percent, and you decrease your heart attack risk by an astounding 20 percent! Now, that's a bargain!

Do not wait for symptoms to appear. In 50 percent of deaths from a heart attack, sudden death was the very first symptom! I strongly urge you to learn your numbers and take the necessary steps to decrease the risk of becoming a mortality statistic of heart disease.

Problem and Prevention

THE VILLAIN

Cholesterol has been in the news almost constantly for several years because it has been firmly identified as the culprit behind heart attacks; finding this villain was most important because heart attacks are the number one cause of death in North America.

The "cholesterol hypothesis" is no longer a hypothesis. "There is no doubt that abnormal cholesterol levels cause morbidity and mortality and that aggressive treatment saves lives." (*Journal of the American Medical Association*, 200: 285: 2508-2509).

We know there are various forms of cholesterol, some bad and some actually good for our hearts. We also know that the ratios among these forms of cholesterol are as important, if not more, as the actual level of cholesterol.

There are even other lipids, namely triglycerides, which come into play as a risk factor.

WHAT IS CHOLESTEROL GOOD FOR ANYWAY?

Well, for one thing, it is the raw material to make sex hormones – not bad to have. It also helps form hormones involved in the stress reaction. A little cholesterol is essential to life because it functions in the transport and communication systems in cell membranes. A lot of cholesterol is converted into bile acids, as much as 90 percent. This is where the plot thickens.

Bile is released by the gall-bladder into the small intestine, near where the food leaves your stomach. Bile helps to digest fats. The enzymes that digest fats are water soluble. Since water and grease do not mix, we need some help. Think of bile like detergent cleaning a dirty plate. Just as the detergent enables water to mix with grease, bile helps to mix fatty foods with water-soluble digestive enzymes.

Here is our problem. There is a lot of cholesterol in bile, and after bile does its job, cholesterol is reabsorbed into the bloodstream further down the small intestine.

Communication is not very good between the liver and the bile in the intestine waiting to be reabsorbed. Consequently, the liver keeps pumping out cholesterol, even though a lot is going to be reabsorbed. If we could stop the reabsorption of the bile acids back into the body, we could make a significant impact on the blood cholesterol. Do you agree? We can stop the reabsorption to a great degree with a little extra calcium and soluble fiber, which we will discuss later.

STOP THE PROBLEM NOW!

Prevention is the only way the epidemic of heart disease can be arrested. We have the knowledge for prevention and that is what I want to share with you in this chapter.

There is no longer any excuse for tolerating heart attack risk factors that are under your control. There are a few people, very few, who have a genetic predisposition for higher cholesterol. These few will need the program I am going to suggest, plus a cholesterol-lowering drug to get levels down to normal.

THE CHALLENGE AND THE PLAN

Here is the challenge. Have your blood lipid profile taken. This is a total analysis of the fats in your blood, including total cholesterol, HDL cholesterol, LDL cholesterol, triglycerides, and some others. From these figures, you can compute some of the ratios I will refer to in this chapter.

After that, start the plan I recommend. Follow this simple plan religiously for four to six weeks. Then have another blood lipid profile done.

In just four to six weeks, your cholesterol level will have dropped by at least 10 percent. That means, if you began at 240 mg/dL, you should be at least down to 215 mg/dL by the end of the challenge time. In some people it drops much more, depending on how high it was at the start. Even more importantly, some other risk factors will improve significantly. The various ratios of lipids, many of which are now considered more important than total cholesterol, will greatly improve. You will have reduced your chances of a heart attack dramatically!

Once you have a little success under your belt, keep to the program until you achieve the optimal numbers. Then, you will be on the way to adding years to your life and life to your years.

Here is the Plan:
- Stop smoking anything (you have to say that nowadays).
- Follow a simple dietary plan.
- Begin an exercise program (with the doctor's okay).
- Drop a few pounds (it's automatic on the plan).
- Take a fiber supplement I will describe.
- Take some extra food supplements and herbs.
- Have another blood lipid profile done.

That's all there is to it! Stick with the program, and your blood lipid profile should continue to improve.

Highlights of the New Cholesterol Guidelines by the US National Cholesterol and Education Program (May 2001)

- People with multiple risk factors for heart disease should keep their LDL less than 100 mg/dL and those with LDL of 130 mg/dL or higher should undergo drug therapy and therapeutic lifestyle changes, which include reduced intake of saturated fats and cholesterol, weight reduction and increased physical activity.

- Type 2 diabetics with high cholesterol should be treated more aggressively whether or not clinical coronary disease is present.

- HDL level of less than 40 mg/dL is considered a risk factor for heart disease, as compared to 35 mg/dL recommended in 1993. A HDL of 60 mg/dL or more is considered protective against heart disease.

- Men and women over 20 years of age should have their total cholesterol, LDL, HDL and triglycerides tested once every five years.

- People with borderline levels of triglycerides are advised to lose weight and exercise. High triglycerides may warrant medication.

- Adults are advised to lower their LDL level through diet before trying medication.

- Lowering LDL can reduce the short term risk of heart disease by as much as 40 percent.

- Foods that contain plant stanols and sterols, or rich in soluble fiber, can boost the diet's LDL-lowering power.

- Hormone Replacement Therapy is not advisable as an alternative to cholesterol-lowering drugs.

The Concern about Cholesterol, HDL, LDL and Triglycerides

AGING CORONARY ARTERIES

We need to lower cholesterol because it is accepted worldwide as the best indicator of the rate your arteries (and you) are aging. To slow that rate, lower your cholesterol and keep it down.

As the artery ages, sludge, gunk, or the scientific word "plaque," deposits in the artery walls. This plaque is mostly cholesterol. It's pretty simple; the higher your cholesterol level, the more rapidly plaque develops in your arteries.

When should you begin to worry? This process can begin with fatty streaks in the artery as young as 11 years of age. If your family has a history of high cholesterol or early death caused by heart attack, have your child's cholesterol checked. This establishes a base line to which you can refer back to in later years.

PLUGGED PLUMBING

Plaque is somewhat like the scale that builds up inside a water pipe. It isn't noticed until the flow of water slows down or the water won't flow at all. A similar event is occurring in your heart's vessels, but you can't handle it as easily as calling a plumber.

As plaque builds, the coronary artery's opening narrows. Because the blood flow is restricted to the heart, you will get shortness of breath on exertion, or even chest pain. This is the way the heart cries out for more oxygen.

The small opening in the artery can be blocked by a blood clot, which stops the flow of the blood. If the blockage is in the small coronary artery, and the tissue death is not extensive, you will have a heart attack and survive. If the blockage is in a large artery, and the heart tissue death is very extensive, you are dead all over.

TYPES OF CHOLESTEROL

As I have said, cholesterol is the culprit that clogs our arteries, but not all cholesterol is created equal. There is bad cholesterol (LDL) and good cholesterol (HDL).

We want LDL to be as low as possible. If your LDL is under 130 mg/dL, that's considered good. If it is over 160 mg/dL, you will be told that this is bad, bad, bad! As for HDL, we obviously want as much as possible. There seems to be an upper limit on how much HDL cholesterol we can produce. It is about 60 mg/dL for men and 80 mg/dL for women. Good numbers to try for are 40+ mg/dL for men and 60+ mg/dL for women.

TC/HDL RATIO

Actually, research has found the ratio of total cholesterol to HDL to be the best predictor of heart disease. You divide the total cholesterol by the HDL. This ratio is perhaps more important than total cholesterol. The mystery about total cholesterol has been this: Why do we see heart attacks in people with fairly low total cholesterol while in others with high cholesterol, no heart attack? Let me give you an example:

	Person A	**Person B**
TOTAL CHOLESTEROL	250 mg/dL	200 mg/dL
HDL	50 mg/dL	20 mg/dL
RATIO	5	10

Person A has a much higher total cholesterol than person B. It would seem that he is in trouble, right? Actually person B with his "normal" cholesterol number is at a much greater risk for a heart attack than person A.

The major difference is the vitally important ratio. Studies have shown that the high ratio in people with low total cholesterol levels is one explanation why a person with low cholesterol will have a heart attack. Person A should get his total cholesterol down because that is still a separate risk factor, but risk-wise, he is in better shape as he has a lower ratio than Person B.

If your cholesterol is over 200 mg/dL, be sure to check the ratio. The normal ratio for men is 4.5 or lower, and for women, 4.0 or lower. Research tells us that 3.5 is good and less than 3.0 is excellent. Several studies support the fact that if you can get your ratio down to between 2.4 and 2.8, you can actually get reversal of heart disease!

TRIGLYCERIDES (FAT)

When you get a blood lipid profile, you will get a number for something called triglycerides. Triglycerides are, for simplification, what we call "fat." When you grab a handful of tummy, love handles, or some other fat storage, you are grabbing triglycerides. Triglycerides are produced in the body from the fats you eat or excess calories coming from alcohol or carbohydrate-rich foods.

Triglycerides come from both animal and plant foods, while cholesterol comes from animal foods only. Triglycerides contain fatty acids while cholesterol does not. Unlike triglycerides, cholesterol does not provide any calories.

High triglycerides are a risk factor to be considered because they are consistently associated with high LDL (the bad kind) and low HDL (the good kind). The mechanism of this association is not well understood, but high triglycerides are considered a heart attack risk factor. An ideal number for triglycerides is less than 125 mg/dL.

When you get your second blood lipid profile at the end of four to six weeks, don't be surprised if your triglycerides are somewhat elevated from the original test. Three things can cause higher triglycerides: a high-fat diet; a high-sugar diet; and weight loss. If you are following the total four-week plan, you will be losing weight slowly. As you lose weight, the fat comes out of the fat cells and into the blood to be removed from the body. Anytime you are on weight loss diet, expect higher than normal triglycerides.

CATCH UP TIME

Let's do a fast summary of the blood lipid profile up to this point, and then get into some more details on cholesterol. There are several numbers that must line up correctly. Remember, each is a separate risk factor. The two most significant are the ratio and total cholesterol.

The Desirable Number Line Up

Total cholesterol:	Less than 200 mg/dL
HDL cholesterol:	More than 40 mg/dL for men
	More than 60 mg/dL for women
LDL cholesterol:	Less than 130 mg/dL
Triglycerides:	Less than 125 mg/dL
Total cholesterol/HDL ratio:	4.5 or lower for men
	4.0 or lower for women

Pay attention, because this is crucial. If just one factor in your lipid profile is abnormal, it is a separate risk factor. For optimal coronary protection, all factors must be in good ranges. Dr. William Castelli of the famous *Framingham Heart Study* says you must know four numbers to stay alive: your total cholesterol, HDL cholesterol, your triglycerides, and your Social Security number.

"If you keep your total cholesterol/HDL ratio under 4.5, your LDL cholesterol under 130 mg/dL, your triglycerides under 125 mg/dL, you exercise, and don't smoke, you will very probably never have a heart attack," says Dr. Castelli. Get your numbers checked now by a good laboratory.

Dietary Control of Cholesterol

THE CHOLESTEROL LOWERING DIET

The diet is basically oriented to reduce saturated fat in your food intake. The National Cholesterol Education Programs Expert Panel (2001) recommends, as the first step of a heart disease prevention diet, to consume less than seven percent of calories from saturated fat and less than 200 mg of dietary cholesterol. It also allows up to 35 percent of daily calories from total fat, provided most of it comes from unsaturated fats, which do not cause a rise in cholesterol levels.

WHY LIMIT SATURATED FATS?

Eating saturated fats can increase cholesterol in your blood more than consuming cholesterol! The chemistry is complex, but it ends with more cholesterol in your blood. So, here are the things to consider:

- Limit red meat to once a week.
- Avoid chicken skin and the fats of meat.
- Avoid processed meat of any kind.
- Watch for hidden fats in deep fried foods, fast foods and processed foods.
- Read labels before you make a purchase.
- Shun foods that are "partially hydrogenated" or "hydrogenated." They contain trans fatty acids (TFA) which raise your LDL cholesterol (bad cholesterol).
- Reduce intake of processed carbohydrates and oily foods.

- Reduce sugar intake and choose foods low in sugar.
- Limit your intake of food with gravies and sauces.
- Avoid or reduce intake of alcohol as it raises your triglycerides.

Good grief, what can I eat? The following is a suggested food plan that we all should follow for good health and maximum energy, even if our cholesterol is normal:

- Eat fowl with skin removed.
- Eat cold water fish at least three times a week. They contain omega-3 fatty acids.
- Eat a variety of colorful vegetables and fruits. They contain vitamins, minerals and phytonutrients such as carotenoids and flavonoids, which contain powerful antioxidants, besides being rich in soluble and insoluble fibers.
- Do less frying; instead bake, boil, poach, broil or steam your food.
- Eat beans and lentils – beware of fat content.
- Eat pasta and oatmeal.
- Eat grains and nuts.
- Drink at least eight glasses of clean purified water.
- Use monounsaturated fats such as olive oil, flaxseed oil, canola and avocado.
- Use fats sparingly. Put less butter on your bread or potato, less salad dressing on your salad and so on.
- Use garlic generously in all your cooking.
- Take spirulina. It is a "superfood." It contains a powerful mix of over 100 organic nutrients including antioxidants, phyto-chemicals, vitamins, minerals, enzymes, GLA, amino acids and chlorophyll; plus, its protein is very similar to human breast milk. Unlike other protein, it is alkali forming and so much akin to fruits and vegetables. Most important of all, it is low in calories and sodium, with no cholesterol or saturated fats.

The US National Cholesterol and Education Program (May 2001) suggests that adults use diet to lower their cholesterol levels before trying medication. The report encourages the consumption of foods rich in soluble fibers such as cereal grains, beans, peas, legumes and a variety of fruits and vegetables to help lower cholesterol levels.

DEAR DIARY

Since our main goal is to reduce saturated fat and limit other fats too, a diet diary is needed. Most of us have no idea how much fat is in the different foods that we eat. I want you to do two things. Buy a book that lists the calories and grams of saturated fat in various foods. Your goal is to keep the saturated fat intake down to below seven percent of your needed calories a day.

The second thing I want you to do is to buy a notebook of some sort in which to keep your diary. Write down everything that goes into your mouth, being sure to keep track of the calories and saturated fat. The diary is to keep us honest and make us very aware of which foods contain the greatest amounts of fat. I call my diary "D.I.E.T." The letters stand for "Did I Eat That?" It keeps me honest!

If you keep up with your food intake and fat grams for four weeks, you will automatically become very discriminating in your food choices. Look at your saturated fat and calories as money in the bank. As you eat each meal, you make withdrawals from your daily fat/calorie account. You only have so much of an allowance to spend, so budget and spend wisely. One person actually kept her diary in a check registry! It was quite effective.

Increase HDL – The "Good Cholesterol"

HDL POWER

Reducing your total cholesterol will definitely lower your heart attack risk. But, raising your HDL will dramatically lower your risk! There are basically five ways to raise your HDL.

Number one, by far, is aerobic exercise. Don't panic! You can count adequate "strolling" among this. Let's do strolling first because it sounds less intimidating.

Researchers at the Cooper Institute for Aerobics Research in Dallas, Texas, concluded that you can raise HDL without vigorous exercise. This study was accepted for publication in the *Journal of the American Medical Association*.

The participants involved 59 healthy women divided into four groups as follows:

GROUP ONE: Walked fast (five miles per hour, almost a run).
GROUP TWO: Walked briskly (four miles an hour).
GROUP THREE: Walked moderately (three miles an hour).
GROUP FOUR: Remained sedentary.

Each walking group covered three miles, five days a week for six months. Results: The first two groups were just about equal in HDL gains, and their aerobic capacities were close. Even the slow walkers got some gain. The only downside of the two slower groups is the time; it took longer to cover the three miles. So, you have a choice: go fast for a shorter period of time or slower for a longer period of time.

Is this really "new" information? No. "Walking is man's best medicine," said Hippocrates in 400 B.C.! It worked then and it will work for you now. Equipment needed: comfortable shoes and a determination to do it!

Raising your HDL is extremely powerful. Several good studies have indicated that you reduce your heart attack risk by an awesome seven percent for each point you elevate your HDLs above 50. It's well worth the rewards to follow all six of the HDL elevating steps.

Exercise your way to health

If you really want to "run up" the good cholesterol, it takes a little more effort. A team led by George Town University researcher Peter Kokkinos, Ph.D., measured cholesterol levels in some 2,900 men, aged 30 to 64. Most were runners; the rest were healthy but sedentary.

When the researchers charted the running mileage and HDL levels, they found that HDL rose by about 0.31 mg/dL for every additional mile that was run. Those who covered the most distance had the highest HDL. The intermediate group had HDL levels 11 percent higher than the non-runners.

Based on the study, researchers recommended the equivalent of running seven to 14 miles a week at a moderate pace. That's about 30 minutes of exercise three to five times a week. Besides walking, aerobic exercise, swimming, biking and racquet games can also help. Remember, it is never too old or too late to start exercising.

Get your weight down to normal or slightly below (BMI 18-24.9)

If you faithfully follow the plan for four to six weeks, your weight will begin to come down automatically. The combination of a low-fat diet and exercise is as close to a sure thing as you can get. Obesity contributes to high cholesterol, high triglycerides and low HDL.

Consume cold water fish

Mackerel, haddock, anchovies, sardines, tuna and some salmon, all contain an unusual fatty acid called eicosapentaenoic acid or EPA for short. The EPA actually lowers triglycerides. As you recall, high

HDL is associated with low triglycerides. This is the reason fish is in your food choices. It's hard to consume as much of these blue skinned fish as you need; there is no "McMackerel," so I recommend an EPA food supplement.

Increase your consumption of soluble fiber
Soluble fiber seems to actually target LDL cholesterol and leave the HDL alone. So, as you lower the total cholesterol in this way, your ratio improves because the HDL stays high or even goes up a point or two.

Do not smoke anything!
This is good advice for anyone. Numerous experts have been asked, "What is the one thing I can do to increase my healthy life span?" The answer is consistent: "Do not smoke." Even second hand smoke may lower HDL.

Get fats out of your diet
About 17 percent of the American diet currently comes from saturated fats. Reducing saturated fat calories to 10 percent of total calories can lower total cholesterol by as much as 20 percent.

Eat more often to lower cholesterol
"If you are already eating well and want to have further benefit, at least for cholesterol, dividing what you eat into more frequent meals may have additional benefits. The more frequently the better – four, five or six (meals) spread out over the day so smaller amounts are eaten more frequently," says Dr. Kay-Tee Khaw of the University of Cambridge. This research is published in *The British Medical Journal*.

A recent guideline on May 15, 2001 by the National Cholesterol Education Program (NCEP) confirm beyond doubt the need for weight control, physical activity and intensified use of nutrition to lower risk of heart disease. Weight control and greater physical activity improves your HDL.

112

Cholesterol-lowering Herbs and Supplements

THE OPTION IS GONE

Food supplements are no longer an option in our diets. There are certain nutrients critically needed to protect us from heart disease and other dreaded killers, such as some forms of cancer. We cannot conveniently get several of these nutrients from our diets in the amounts needed for protection. One nutrient, vitamin E, is impossible to obtain in adequate amounts. Supplements are essential!

SOLUBLE FIBER SUPPLEMENT

A fiber supplement is a key player in our heart disease prevention program.

This may amaze you: a soluble fiber supplement will reduce cholesterol for most people even if they do nothing else. Why do I recommend a supplement? This is because even those who eat a very well-balanced diet do not get enough of the key soluble fibers in their day-to-day diets.

I have read an excellent study concerning a supplement with four fibers. The study was headed by Dr. William Haskell of the Stanford University School of Medicine. The results of the study were reported in the *American Journal of Cardiology*. The researchers used a combination of pectin, psyllium husks, guar, and locust bean gums.

In one part of the study, the soluble supplement was combined with weight loss and exercise, just as what we recommend. The results were phenomenal. In just four weeks, the total cholesterol of the participants was reduced by an average of 15 percent and LDL cholesterol was reduced by 22 percent!

Remember, for each one percent drop in total cholesterol, you reduce your heart attack risk by two percent. The results of this study represent an amazing decrease in heart attack risk of 30 percent! Is this a lot? Yes! These results are even better than some of the LDL cholesterol lowering drugs on the market, and without the side effects!

How Does This Work?
Cholesterol once made, cannot be broken down. It can only be removed from our body in the form of bile acids and cholesterol molecules.

Soluble fiber can bind bile acids (they contain up to 95 percent cholesterol) in the small intestine to prevent them from being reabsorbed! It holds them and takes them to elimination. Not only that, these fibers zero in on LDL and leave the good HDL alone. In addition to soluble fiber, extra calcium in the gut combines with fats to form soaps, which the body cannot reabsorb. The impact of calcium is not near that of soluble fiber, but every little bit helps.

The best time to take the supplement is just before your largest meal of the day. This meal will stimulate the most bile acid release from your gall bladder. You take the supplement first because you want these little cholesterol-binding sponges to be ahead of the food, ready to trap the cholesterol-rich bile. I would also take the supplement just before one other meal of the day. Studies indicate you need to take it at least twice a day for best results. If your cholesterol is really resistant, go to three servings a day for awhile.

There are two cautions to observe when you add fiber, be it from your diet or through supplements. First, add it slowly so your body can adjust to the additional fiber. If added too rapidly, it can produce gas. Also, be sure you get 8 to 10 glasses of purified water a day. Water helps fiber do its various jobs better.

MULTI-VITAMIN/MINERAL

The first supplement to add to your daily food regime should be a multi-vitamin/mineral preparation. Personally, I feel everyone should be taking a multi. Numerous studies show that we do not get all the nutrients we need in necessary amounts.

No recognized vitamin or mineral in the Daily Value (DV) has been shown to have an adverse effect on your blood lipids, even if consumed slightly above the recommended levels. On the other hand, a shortage of some of these has been shown to put some of the lipid factors out of balance. A good general multi is just insurance for those nutrients that may be missing from your day-to-day diet.

EICOSAPENTAENOIC ACID (EPA) – AN OMEGA-3 FATTY ACID

We have known for years that native Eskimos who consume large quantities of blue-skinned, cold-water fish have lower incidences of coronary heart disease. At first, this was just dismissed as genetics peculiar to this group. Then, some of these native Eskimos began consuming the American diet. Interestingly enough, they began to develop the same heart attack problems as we have.

We owe a lot of credit to a Danish epidemiologist by the name of Jorn Dyerberg. He made a careful study of the heart attack occurrences among Danes (who eat a diet like ours) and Greenland Eskimos (who eat a diet high in EPA). Heart disease is the number one killer of both Danes and North Americans, but note the differences between these population groups and the Eskimos. The heart attack rate among North Americans is around 46 *percent* but the heart attack rate among Greenland Eskimos is less than *eight percent* ... a startling *38 percent difference!* How does EPA do this?

Benefits
EPA "thins out" the blood. Through this process, there are fewer

tendencies for the blood to develop clots, which can clog the vessels and cause a heart attack. Remember, in 90+ percent of heart attacks, a blood clot is the cause.

For most people, it will lower triglycerides, if high. High triglycerides are associated with low HDL (the good kind). If you can get your triglycerides down, it often results in the HDL moving up into a more healthy range.

It has, in some cases, even had a positive effect on high blood pressure. The mechanism of this is not understood. It could result from a slight widening of the blood vessels, or it could be due to the fact that EPA makes the blood more "slippery," causing it to flow more smoothly.

As a blood clot begins to form, one of the early stages is a clumping of the little cells that initiate the clot and the formation of tiny threads called fibrin. These pre-clots can cause blockage in blood vessels. EPA actually helps to dissolve these clots (fibrinolysis) before they develop into a true, life-threatening clot.

One caution: If you are taking a blood thinning drug, consult with your physician before talking EPA. The supplement could interfere with the drug.

GARLIC

In the past, the cry from the scientific community has been, "There's not enough evidence. Show us that garlic can stand up to scientific testing." Today, a growing number of researchers are taking up this challenge. Here are a few of the results.

In a large study of 220 patients, the garlic group took 800 mg of powdered garlic for four months. This group experienced a 12 percent drop in cholesterol and a 17 percent drop in triglycerides. The placebo group had little change.

In Germany, where garlic is a licensed medicine for atherosclerosis, a study came out of Munich University. Patients were put on a low-fat diet, and the cholesterol fell 10 percent and stabilized. Garlic was added, and the cholesterol fell another 10 percent.

In a survey of dozens of studies, the results were remarkably consistent. With garlic, you can expect a drop in cholesterol of anywhere from 10 to 20 percent. It doesn't take much to do the job. In one study, 261 people were given 800 mg of dried garlic for 16 weeks. That is about the equivalent of a small clove of fresh garlic. There was an average drop of 10 percent in cholesterol.

A SOY PROTEIN SUPPLEMENT

You may have heard that North Americans consume too much protein. That information came from studies in the late 1970s and early 1980s, before we were told to take the vital health step of cutting down on fat, especially saturated fat. The problem is that most of our usual protein sources (meat, milk, cheese) have a lot of fat attached to them. As you lower the fat, you automatically lower the protein.

Susan Potter, Ph.D., at the University of Illinois at Urbana-Champaign, studied soy protein and heart disease. In testing various soy products and combinations, she found that isolated soy protein worked the best, resulting in a 12 percent drop in total cholesterol and an 11.5 percent drop in LDL.

The researchers concluded: "The fact that a significant reduction is obtained by consuming only 50 grams a day of soy protein, sets a practical and achievable goal that would be beneficial in the treatment of high blood cholesterol and coronary artery disease." In follow-up studies by Dr. Potter's group, it was shown that even 25 grams (roughly one-half cup) of soy protein daily could result in significant reduction of cholesterol levels in those with elevated levels.

To put all of these in a nutshell, a paper was recently published in the *New England Journal of Medicine* summarizing the findings of 38 well-controlled studies on soy protein and cholesterol. Overall, there was about a 9 percent reduction in total cholesterol and nearly a 13 percent reduction in the bad LDL.

How Does Soy Protein Work?

The buildup of plaque in arteries is thought to be caused by something that creates damage or alteration to the cells lining the coronary arteries. Many researchers now strongly believe this injury may involve oxidation of LDL caused by free radicals.

We know cholesterol, specifically LDL cholesterol, is the culprit. Here is how it all works. Certain cells in the body are garbage disposal units. They line blood vessels and when something that does not belong in the blood vessels floats by; they grab it and eat it. These cells are called macrophages. "Macro" means big and "phage" means eater.

The "big eaters" consume the oxidized LDL cholesterol quite well, but the problem is, they can't digest it. These cells become packed with fat and are called "foam cells." They become so stuffed that they cause the artery to bulge out into the lumen, the passageway of the artery. This protrusion attracts other cell debris, and we have the beginning of a fibrous bulging plaque that can cut off the flow of blood. Antioxidants help prevent the initial step – oxidation of the LDL.

A team of researchers from the Hirosaki University School of Medicine recently tested this theory on animals. They divided rabbits into two groups. Both received the same diet, but one group was given soy protein and the other Probucol, a prescribed drug known to be an antioxidant.

In both groups the oxidation rate fell rapidly. In fact, the soy worked even better than the drug, Probucol, in preventing LDL oxidation! The results of the study were published in the *Annals of the New York Academy of Sciences*. "Thus, because soy proteins decreased the production of oxidized and deformed LDL, they are very useful in preventing the development of atherosclerotic diseases," said the authors of the study.

Still another way soy may help prevent heart problems is its amino acid composition. Although it is equal to meat and eggs as a complete protein, it has a different amino acid profile. Soy protein is lower in two essential amino acids (lysine and methionine) than meat. Studies have shown that when lysine is added to a soy diet, LDL levels can rise. Therefore, the ratio of the amino acids in soy may help prevent the formation of plaque.

The mechanism of just exactly how soy works its magic with cholesterol will be the subject of many studies. However, the main point to make is that soy works and works quite well!

VITAMIN E IS A MUST!

I routinely take a vitamin E food supplement, and I am careful to never miss a day. The research is too compelling. Vitamin E is an extremely powerful antioxidant and works especially well with cholesterol. We have covered the mechanics of LDL, oxidants and the artery clogging process under soy protein, so let's take a look at the research on vitamin E.

Dr. Daniel Steinberg of the University of California at San Diego led a most revealing experiment. The scientists mixed LDL with macrophages in a test tube. In spite of their efforts, they could not force the macrophages to take up the LDL very quickly. Then they oxidized the LDL. "The macrophages took up the LDL three to 10 times faster," said Steinberg.

When they added vitamin E (a strong antioxidant) to the same mix, the LDL was protected from being taken up by the macrophages. What a great discovery! If LDL isn't engulfed by macrophages, it cannot clog your arteries. This study was reported in the *Journal of the American Medical Association*. It has since been confirmed by numerous reports.

An ongoing Harvard University study headed by Dr. Meir J. Stampfer reported on 87,000 female nurses. Those who took a supplement of vitamin E each day had about one-third less risk of heart attack or death from coronary disease than those who did not take supplements.

The Harvard study even made a believer out of the researcher. Dr. Stampfer of the Harvard School of Public Health in Boston began the 87,000 nurse study expecting to disprove the idea that vitamin E could reduce the risk. He says: "It just didn't seem plausible that a simple maneuver like taking vitamin E would have such a profound effect."

This next study is extremely interesting. Last year, researchers reported evidence that the level of antioxidants in the blood may have more influence on heart disease than do classic coronary risk factors. In a comparison of 16 European populations of men, they found that a low vitamin E level was more closely related to the development of heart disease, than high blood cholesterol and high blood pressure!

THE BATTLE CONTINUES WITH VITAMIN C

Several studies have shown that in populations where vitamin C intake is low, heart disease deaths are high, and where vitamin C intake is high, heart disease deaths are low.

Dr. Ishwarlal Jialal has done some work on vitamin C. He recently reported on the power of vitamin C as an antioxidant in the journal *Atherosclerosis*. Dr. Jialal did a study very similar to the one Dr. Steinberg did with vitamin E. The results were astounding. Vitamin C cut the macrophage absorption of LDL by 93 percent! Jialal noted that smoking, diabetes and stress deplete the body's vitamin C. "All three are risk factors for heart disease, lending credence to the theory that oxidation plays a crucial role in the development of atherosclerosis," he said.

How does all this fit together? How can vitamin E and C do the same thing? I think this may be the answer. Vitamin E is a fat-soluble vitamin and works on reducing oxidation in the fatty parts of the cells. Vitamin C is a water-soluble vitamin and works in the watery or aqueous parts of the cell. Both have a similar effect, but they just work in different cellular areas. If this is true, it would mean they have a complementary effect on each other.

In May of 1992, University of California, Los Angeles researchers reported on a huge study of 11,000 Americans. They found that increasing intake of vitamin C nearly halves the death rate from heart disease and lengthens life expectancy by up to six years.

More good news is that vitamin C is safe even at high levels of intake. When Linus Pauling began his vitamin C revolution, he was advocating 5,000 to 10,000 mg a day. These recommendations caused scientists to conduct numerous studies on the safety of vitamin C. The literature supports the safety of 5,000 to 10,000 mg a day.

BETA-CAROTENE CUTS HEART PROBLEMS BY HALF

That was the title of an article on beta-carotene which is a form of pro-vitamin A. It is the nutrient that gives deep colored vegetables and fruits their distinctive hues.

The results of this ongoing study were reported in the *Medical Tribune*. A total of 22,000 men were split into two groups. One group took 50 mg (83,000 IU) of beta-carotene every other day and the other group a placebo. At the end of six years, the beta-carotene group had half as many "major cardiovascular events" such as heart attack or stroke. Half of these men were also taking aspirin. It is from this study that the idea originated to give aspirin to heart risk patients.

Beta-carotene could help slow the progress of heart disease. For instance, in one study, 333 men had signs of heart disease, stable angina, bypass surgery or angioplasty. None of the 333 men who took beta-carotene and aspirin had a heart attack. Do they work together? If you want to try the aspirin, discuss it with your physician first.

Beta-carotene is another one of those safe nutrients to take. If you took a lot, your skin would turn an orange color; that's the only side effect. The major studies all seem to focus on an average of 80,000 IU every other day. That would mean five cups of spinach, or two cups of carrots, or 25 cups of broccoli. I like all of these vegetables, but just not that much. I definitely choose to add a beta-carotene food supplement.

B COMPLEX

There are eight members of the B complex, all of which work together like a family. Each helps the other do a better job. Much of the B complex is very fragile and can be destroyed by storage, shipping and cooking. The big three killers of the complex are heat, air and light. For instance, prolonged heating can destroy up to 40 percent of the thiamin in a serving of green beans.

Various members of the B complex have been shown to lower blood cholesterol, lower triglycerides, increase the good HDLs, and expand or widen the blood vessels. Granted, these effects are very small in most cases, but I want all the help I can get. However, some members of the B complex, such a folic acid, offer some really significant heart disease protection.

Folic acid is extremely vital in preventing heart disease. A by-product of metabolism called homocysteine can build up in the body and increase the risk of heart disease. *The New England Journal of Medicine* reported that people with high levels of homocysteine were 30 times more likely to develop vascular disease than those with normal levels.

To put these numbers in perspective, high homocysteine is a more potent risk factor than high cholesterol, high blood pressure, or cigarette smoking! Here is the good news: Folic acid can protect us from homocysteine.

Extra B complex is a must for those over 55. As you age, the B complex is not absorbed as efficiently as when you were younger. As a result, you require a greater concentration of B's for better absorption.

Always add the entire B complex even if you are after the beneficial effects of just one member such as folic acid. Remember, the B complex works as a team, each helping and balancing the other.

CALCIUM

If you decide to become a vegetarian, all of the familiar sources of calcium are eliminated. On the food plan suggested, you are going to be reducing dairy products to only those with a low-fat content. Some people complain of the somewhat "flat" taste of low-and-non-fat-dairy. Others (some 26 percent) cannot tolerate the lactose in many dairy products. We need over 1,000 mg of calcium, but the sad truth is Americans only average about 660 mg. All this tells me that nearly all Americans need a calcium supplement for optimal health.

Calcium excretion via the bowel has been shown to be beneficial to our heart. We know how soluble fiber binds cholesterol and takes it to elimination; well, calcium gives us more help here. It combines with cholesterol and other fats such a triglycerides and form soap-like compounds. The body cannot reabsorb these compounds, so they are excreted.

Calcium has also been shown to help lower blood pressure in about 26 percent of those with the problem. This is about the same percentage of people who are sodium sensitive, so there may be some connection.

LECITHIN

This accessory nutrient has been shown to be of benefit in lowering cholesterol. A 16-week study at the Rutgers Medical School showed a "marked decrease in serum cholesterol." A Belgian study of some 100 patients showed a 40 percent drop in cholesterol. In both of those studies, the cholesterol was high to begin with.

Lecithin does its work in an enzyme system called LCAT or lecithin cholesterol acetyl transferase. Without going into complex details, cholesterol production is reduced through this system.

HAWTHORN (Crataegus oxyacantha)

Recent research shows that oxidized LDL cholesterol and not just LDL cholesterol is a villain that causes clogged arteries and heart attacks.

Hawthorn helps reduce cholesterol in the following way:

*   It contains a powerful antioxidant "oligometric proanthocynidins," that helps prevent oxidization of LDL cholesterol in the blood. This process prevents the building up of plaque on the arterial wall (atherosclerosis).

*   It helps promote the conversion of LDL cholesterol into HDL (good) cholesterol (Rister R., *Japanese Herbal Medicine*, Avery 1999, p. 60).

*   It prevents cholesterol from accumulating in the liver by encouraging production of cholesterol-laden bile, which passes into the intestine and out of the body.

GUGULIPID (Commiphora mukul)

Gugulipid is a patented extract of gugul (mukul myrrh tree), containing 2.5 percent guggulsterones, its active compound. The word "gugul" means "gummy resins." It is an Indian Ayurvedic medicine that has a history of at least 3,000 years.

In both human and animal studies, gugulipid helps lower total cholesterol, LDL and triglycerides and raise HDL cholesterol, although most studies are small.

In the United States, a similar story is told: "Significant cholesterol and triglycerides reduction," says Richard Conaut, author of *Natural Alternatives for Lowering Cholesterol and Triglycerides*.

If you are on cholesterol-lowering drugs, please consult your doctor before taking gugulipid. Research shows that it is non-toxic and safe to take.

WRAP UP

Let's wrap this discussion up and give a summary to be sure you are on the right track to controlling your cholesterol. Remember, we had two things: a challenge and a plan.

Here is the challenge:
Have your blood lipid profile taken. This is a total analysis of the fats in your blood including total cholesterol, HDL cholesterol, LDL cholesterol and triglycerides. From these figures, you can compute the ratios I referred to earlier. Know your numbers! Are you headed for a heart attack – or will you escape?

Here is the plan:
- Stop smoking anything.
- Begin an exercise program. *The Aerobics Program For Total Well-Being* by Dr. Kenneth Cooper is an excellent book for guidance in exercise.
- Drop a few pounds.
- Take a soluble-fiber supplement.
- Follow the simple dietary plan.
- Take some extra food supplements and herbs.
- Then after four to six weeks, have another blood lipid profile done. I believe you will be pleasantly surprised.

CLOSING REMARKS

If healthy lifestyle and nutrition cannot help you lower your cholesterol level, drugs may be the only alternative. However, you must continue to practice healthy living along with a proper diet and nutrition.

Generally, there are four major groups of cholesterol-lowering drugs in use:

- Statins (HMG CoA reductase)
- Resins (bile acid sequestrants)
- Fibrates (fibric acid derivatives)
- Niacin (nicotinic acid).

Your doctor will be the best person to advise you on which cholesterol-lowering drug would be suitable for you.

7

THE HIGH BLOOD PRESSURE CONNECTION

Understanding High Blood Pressure

YOUR ODDS AGAINST HIGH BLOOD PRESSURE

You may not have it now, but you probably will. By about age 60, six out of 10 Americans have blood pressure that is high enough to require treatment. If you live long enough, you will most likely get high blood pressure. Only a small minority of Americans escape this condition.

The tragedy is that many do not even know they have it. High blood pressure (hypertension) has very few symptoms until it is too late. It is indeed a silent killer, but it is not inevitable. Among the risk factors for stroke and heart disease, it is one of the most preventable.

No one actually dies of high blood pressure. They die of other illnesses brought on or made much worse by high blood pressure. These include stroke, heart attack, heart failure, angina, kidney failure and many others. This "silent killer within" also detracts from our quality of life by causing headaches, depression, fainting spells, ringing in the ears and loss of eyesight.

Here is the good news! Nearly 90 percent of high blood pressure can be controlled with diet, food supplements and other lifestyle modifications. But, like most things in life, the choice is yours. You can choose not to have your blood pressure checked and live in the dark, or you can have it checked about twice a year and at least know where you stand. Even if your blood pressure is acceptable now, this chapter will give you ways to prevent, or at least delay the occurrence of high blood pressure.

If it is found that you have high blood pressure, take heart. Most can be controlled without drugs – if you are willing to make the necessary choices. The lifestyle changes are well worth the effort

129

because you can avoid the unpleasant side effects caused by most high blood pressure medications. This will give you a healthier, richer and happier life.

BLOOD PRESSURE

As the heart pumps, the vessels most affected are the arteries. Pressure in the arteries is our "blood pressure." Blood pressure is read as two numbers: systolic and diastolic (both from Greek words meaning contract and relax, respectively). Systolic pressure is generated when your heart muscle contracts and forcefully sends the blood through the arteries. The diastolic pressure is the remaining pressure in the arteries while the heart is refilling and getting ready to beat again.

Blood pressure is expressed in millimeters of mercury (mm Hg). Until recently, instruments with a glass column of mercury were used in the measurement of blood pressure. These devices are very accurate, but a bit cumbersome. They have given way to the convenience of aneroid dials. If your systolic pressure is 120 and your diastolic is 80, it would be written as 120/80 or spoken as "one-twenty over eighty."

THE MEASUREMENT

A rubber cuff is attached to your upper arm. It is then pumped up to above your systolic blood pressure. A valve on the pump allows the pressure to slowly be released while the doctor listens to an artery in your arm. At first he hears nothing, but as he releases more air from the cuff, he will hear a thump. This is the first heart sound and marks your systolic blood pressure. The doctor will continually hear thumps as more air released; then the sound changes to the swishing noise. Pressure at this sound is the diastolic pressure.

We have come a long way since the old mercury columns.

Now blood pressure can be measured electronically. These machines also give you pulse rate. These sophisticated devices are available in most drugstores. Many drugstores and pharmacy outlets have devices mounted near the prescription counter. You can use these to get a free reading. I would not trust a free drugstore reading to be totally accurate, but if you get a high reading, have it double checked by a professional.

Both the systolic and diastolic pressures are recorded as "mm Hg" (millimeters of mercury). The recording represents how high the mercury column is raised by the pressure that matches your blood pressure.

WHAT CAUSES HIGH BLOOD PRESSURE (HYPERTENSION)?

Some populations in other countries never get hypertension – until they move to our country and develop our lifestyle. Thus, many researchers relate the problem to diet, stress and other lifestyle factors which we will cover.

Most of the time, high blood pressure is called essential hypertension or primary hypertension. This means, in medical jargon, the absolute cause is not known. Essential hypertension accounts for 85 to 90 percent of all cases. This type of high blood pressure often seems to run in families. As much as 40 percent of those with high blood pressure have immediate family members with the problem. About 23 percent of Americans are salt-sensitive and need to drastically curb their salt intake.

There is no cure for hypertension, but it can be controlled. Hold that thought for a second. If we can control hypertension, then we can also prevent it in the first place, can't we?

There are a number of lifestyle factors that influence high blood pressure, but do not directly cause it. The choices you can make to prevent and control high blood pressure are the subjects of this chapter.

The other form of high blood pressure is called secondary

hypertension. This means that the high blood pressure is caused by some other conditions. This can be a hormone imbalance, a tumor of some regulatory organ, or kidney problems. By controlling or curing the basic problem, secondary hypertension may just disappear.

HOW HIGH IS HIGH?

Physicians used to talk about "borderline" or "mild" hypertension, defined as beginning around 140/90. But the language is false and misleading. An example is pregnancy. You can't be "borderline" or "mildly" pregnant! We now have some new terms classifying hypertension in stages. However, even "high normal" calls for some immediate lifestyle changes and monitoring.

You should get an accurate check of your blood pressure at least once a year, regardless of your age. If your blood pressure is above normal, see the chart for guidelines. If you have a family history of heart disease or hypertension, you may need more frequent monitoring. Remember, the disease is, for the most part, silent. Your blood pressure can get very high before symptoms are noticeable. Some people do experience symptoms, but often ignore them as "nothing to worry about."

The following table gives you some guidelines.

How Blood Pressure Is Defined

CATEGORY	SYSTOLIC/DIASTOLIC	RECOMMENDATION
Normal	Less than 130/85	Recheck in two years.
High Normal	130-139/85-89	Recheck in one year; begin lifestyle modifications.

CATEGORY	SYSTOLIC/DIASTOLIC	RECOMMENDATION
Hypertension		
Stage 1	140-159/90-99	Confirm in two months; begin lifestyle modifications.
Stage 2	160-179/100-109	Medical evaluation; begin treatment within one month.
Stage 3	180-209/110-119	Medical evaluation; begin treatment within one week.
Stage 4	210/120 and over	Immediate medical evaluation and treatment.

SOME COMMON SYMPTOMS OF HIGH BLOOD PRESSURE

The symptoms listed below may be very mild or start very slowly. Of course, some never get these symptoms at all, and no one gets all of them. If you are aware of several of these symptoms in your life, it might not be a bad idea to get your blood pressure checked.

The most common symptoms are:
- Fainting spells
- Blurred vision
- Tension when there is no cause
- Flushing or redness of the face
- Spontaneous nosebleeds
- Morning headaches
- Ringing in the ears
- Depression without apparent cause
- Unexplained dizziness

These are all early warning signs and should be heeded by simply having your blood pressure checked. The biggest early warning signal of all is a Transient Ischemic Attack (TIA) which occurs before one-half of all strokes.

TRANSIENT ISCHEMIC ATTACK (TIA)

A TIA is a brief "mini stroke" that temporarily reduces the blood supply to the brain. Each year, over 50,000 people suffer a TIA. Often, the symptoms are so fleeting that they are dismissed, but a TIA is a very serious warning sign. Within five years of a TIA, 35 percent develop a full-blown stroke!

This brief interruption of blood to the brain produces stroke-like symptoms with little or no permanent damage. Some of the symptoms are weakness, tingling, or numbness in the arms and legs on one or both sides of the body, vision and language problems, confusion, vertigo, poor balance or lack of coordination.

The onset of a TIA is usually sudden and often quite brief. While a few episodes can last up to 24 hours, most pass in a few minutes, and nearly all resolve within an hour. Of the TIAs that last more than an hour, about 86 percent develop into full-blown strokes.

A TIA is usually the result of a small clot breaking loose in an artery that leads to the brain. The clot comes to an opening in the artery that is too small to get through, and it lodges there. Some blood still flows around the partial blockage, but not enough to feed the brain properly. The situation resolves itself when the clot finally slips through or the body's clot dissolving enzymes reopen the artery.

If you have a TIA, get help immediately. Do not dismiss your symptoms because they have stopped. You have just had a wake-up call that a bomb is about to go off in your head. In fact, about five percent of those who have a TIA will have a stroke within a month of the initial episode.

Of course, the most effective way to avoid symptoms of high

blood pressure and TIAs is to control blood pressure in the first place. Even a reading of high-normal (130-139/85-89) increases stroke risk by around 50 percent!

TWO BASIC TYPES OF STROKE

The most common type of stroke is the thrombic stroke. This could be called a heart attack in the brain. The blood vessels supplying blood to the brain become narrowed due to the buildup of fatty plaque. The plaque-lined blood vessel becomes abruptly and totally blocked by a blood clot. The impact can be sudden and deadly, like a bullet. Instantaneous and complete weakness or paralysis may strike one side of your body, speech may be disrupted and, in severe cases, you may lapse into a deep coma.

The least common stroke is the hemorrhagic stroke. It causes spontaneous bleeding into the brain from the rupture of an aneurysm. Picture an inner tube being inflated. One part of the tube is weak and begins to bulge out from the rest of tube. As the air pressure increases, the bulge gets larger and finally bursts. You just had a ruptured aneurysm of your inner tube. These aneurysms develop from years of high blood pressure slowly weakening the blood vessels.

High blood pressure is the number one risk factor for a stroke of any kind. Death from stroke is number three just behind heart disease and cancer. A sustained increase of blood pressure about 20 percent over normal increases your chances of a stroke three-fold. If you have long-standing, untreated hypertension, then your chances increase to seven times greater than someone with normal pressure.

If the risk of a stroke isn't enough to encourage you to make some changes in your life and prevent high blood pressure, consider some of the other side effects.

OTHER PROBLEMS OF HIGH BLOOD PRESSURE

Silent and relentlessly, high blood pressure wears out and ages the large and small arteries of your body. Your blood vessels are actually degenerating. The heart begins to grow in size to try to push blood against the pressure, and at the same time it begins to tire out. Congestive heart failure is on the way. Your kidneys will scar and shrink. The retina of your eyes may become damaged, leading to loss of sight. Fatty deposits increasingly line your artery walls. High blood pressure is a prime risk factor for a heart attack.

Under the circumstances, it would be advisable for people between 25 and 30 of age to have their blood pressure checked once a year and those above 40 should do it at least twice a year.

Now, if having read this far, you are still not convinced you need to do something to help prevent high blood pressure, blow on a mirror to see if it fogs. If it doesn't, you are already dead! High blood pressure is extremely dangerous, and we need to take action now!

Dietary Changes

THE RATIO OF POTASSIUM TO SODIUM (K-FACTOR)

There are four risk factors for high blood pressure that stand out from all the rest: an extremely strong genetic tendency; excessive alcohol intake; overweight; and too much sodium with too little potassium.

The ratio of potassium to sodium is one common denominator of high blood pressure. Divide the potassium in a food by the sodium. The resultant number is the K-factor. If a particular food contains 300 mg of potassium and 100 mg of sodium, it has a K-factor of three, which is good.

Potassium is found mostly inside the cells, and sodium is in the fluid that bathes the outside of the cells. In fact, inside each cell is a sodium pump to keep the sodium out. These two minerals along with the chloride are called electrolytes. Pure water does not transmit electricity, but water containing these salts does. This is the key to nerve transmission in the body. Nature's balance between the potassium inside the cell and the sodium outside the cell should be a ratio of three or higher. The body works very hard to maintain this balance and unloading excess sodium is where our high blood pressure problem starts.

WHY DOES THE BODY RETAIN WATER?

Suppose the body realizes it has too much sodium and wants to dump some through the kidneys whose very job is to conserve that sodium. The body has two ways to do this: both involve an increase in blood pressure.

First, it constricts the blood vessels and increases the pressure to the kidneys. This pressure forces more sodium through the kidney's recovery filter. But, you see, to get rid of the excess sodium, the blood pressure has to be raised.

The second way to get rid of sodium is to retain water, dilute the sodium, and cause the kidney to excrete both water and sodium. The problem is that the increased volume of retained water in our closed blood vessel system raises the blood pressure.

Both of these mechanisms work together. The net result is an increase in blood pressure as the body works to get back to the proper potassium/sodium ratio. This is the only way the body knows. Here is the terminal problem: If this elevation takes place often enough, the blood volume stays increased, the vascular system adapts, and normal blood pressure slowly increases until hypertension is the end result.

QUICK SUMMARY

If the potassium/sodium ratio gets far below three, the blood pressure will go up. A ratio of three or higher protects the body from high blood pressure to an amazing degree. We don't know all of the exact mechanisms of this potassium/sodium ratio connection but we do know for sure that three and above is what the body requires to control blood pressure. This ratio seems to maintain the desirable balance of potassium inside the cells to the proper balance of sodium outside the cells. Eating a diet lower in sodium and higher in potassium is in harmony with nature and will maintain the proper balance of your body chemistry.

SPEAKING OF SALT

Some people with high blood pressure are salt-sensitive. Experts vary in their estimates from 20 to 50 percent. Salt-sensitive people can tolerate only a very little bit of salt before their pressure goes up. At around 500 mg or about 1/8 teaspoon, they are in trouble. If you have high blood pressure, go on a very low-salt diet and see if it helps. If you have mild hypertension, and you couple salt reduction with weight loss, you can usually lower your medication or get completely off it.

DIETARY CHANGES

- Do not salt your food. About 75 percent of the salt in your food is already added by the manufacturer. Watch for hidden salt in food. Read food labels.
- Instead of using salt, become creative with herbs and spices.
- Eat no processed meat products! This includes luncheon meats, hot dogs, and processed poultry.
- Do not use canned or frozen vegetables. In the processing, the K-factor is lowered.
- Do not eat processed foods unless you know both the potassium and sodium content. The potassium must be at least twice the sodium.
- If you must, have only one alcoholic drink a day.
- Avoid fried foods and skin of fowl and fats of meat.
- Stay out of fast food restaurants; there is nothing there for you except temptation.
- Limit caffeine-containing products.
- Avoid refined carbohydrates. Sugars and alcohol do not supply nutrients. In fact, they rob vital nutrients from the body.
- If possible, stay away from food chemicals such as preservatives, coloring and other additives. A good rule of thumb is this: If it won't rot, don't buy it.
- Watch out for hidden fats in your food.

FOODS FOR PEOPLE WITH HIGH BLOOD PRESSURE

- For dessert, learn to enjoy fresh fruit. As a rule, baked foods such as pies and cakes are too high in sodium.
- Eat a variety of colorful fruits and veggies; however, wash them

thoroughly to get rid of the pesticides present before cooking them. They contain phytonutrients such as flavonoids and carotenoids with known or unknown blood pressure lowering compounds.

- The diet should be low in fat and high in fiber.
- Low-fat dairy products are fine.
- Eat a diet low in red meat. Think of red meat as something you add to a dish rather than the main dish.
- Fowl with skin removed is good.
- Have clean, uncontaminated, cold-water fish such as salmon, mackerel and sardine at least three times a week. They contain omega-3 fatty acids.
- Beans and lentils are excellent.
- Add grains and nuts to your diet.
- Eat foods rich in potassium. You can get that from vegetables, nuts, soy beans, fish, potatoes and bananas.
- Chew on celery stalks. Coumarin found in celery, helps lower blood pressure.
- Use garlic and onions generously in your cooking.
- Consume foods rich in calcium such as yogurt, tofu, canned sardines, salmon and leafy green vegetables (kale, broccoli, collard greens and turnip).
- Use olive and monounsaturated oil for your cooking.
- Whenever possible, boil, steam, broil, or stir fry your food; never add salt.

Some of these changes may be totally at odds with the way you are accustomed to eating. But remember, the way you currently eat got you where you are now! Eat food for health instead of just for taste.

Making these healthy dietary changes is a giant step on the road to not only reducing blood pressure, but lowering weight, preventing a number of cancers, preventing heart disease and increasing your energy. When you sit down to eat, look at the food and ask yourself a question: Will this food improve and promote health or will it destroy my health and well being?

Change Your Lifestyle

BIRTH CONTROL PILLS

The "pill" can raise your systolic pressure a little, by about five points, and the diastolic pressure, two points. This elevation is generally not significant. In rare cases, a woman will develop persistent elevations that require stopping the pill, but for most, the small elevation brought on by the pill is acceptable – unless you smoke!

SMOKING

I think by now most of us realize that, contrary to what the tobacco people have told us for years, smoking is not good for us in any form or fashion. The longest running heart study in America, the *Framingham Study*, found that smoking doubled the risk of stroke. *The Nurses Health Study* reported that women who smoke two packs a day are at four times the risk. Women who use oral contraceptives and also smoke have 40 times the risk of stroke compared to those who neither smoke nor use oral contraceptives.

Smoking causes the blood vessels to constrict, thus raising the blood pressure. For some reason, smoking specifically constricts the main artery to the kidney. Coupled with an increase in blood pressure, this can really set you up for some bad kidney problems.

Here is the good news! Just five years after you stop smoking, your stroke risk will become the same as someone who has never smoked in his or her life! By not buying cigarettes, you have eliminated what many believe to be the most significant health-risk factor in your life – and you will have saved nearly US$12,000. Name one drug at any price that can produce those kinds of results! Stop smoking now!

ALCOHOL

Limit your intake to one drink a day. That's 1.5 ounces of 80-proof, five ounces of wine, or 12 ounces of beer. All contain about the same amount of alcohol. "Blood pressure is exquisitely sensitive to alcohol," says Johns Hopkins' Paul Whelton. "The evidence is consistent and powerful."

You don't have to quit entirely. "It's only those who drink more than two alcoholic beverages a day who will substantially raise their risk for high blood pressure," says Dr. William Haskell of Stanford University.

For some reason, the older you are, the more effect alcohol has on your blood pressure. A study of 4,783 men and women found that those in their 20s who consumed two "shots" a day had a "modest but consistent" increase in pressure.

Those 35 and older, drinking the same amount, were twice as likely to be classified as hypertensive. If you are over 50 and have high blood pressure, try abstaining for awhile and see if it goes down.

STRESS

The bad news is that people with essential hypertension show an exaggerated blood pressure increase in response to stress. The good news is, these same people also have a greater response to blood-pressure-lowering relaxation exercise as well. Such individuals are called hot reactors and have to be particularly careful in stressful situations which can raise already elevated blood pressure.

Frustration, worry, anxiety, pressure, emotional turmoil and deadlines are all normal human reactions to perceived traumatic events that life deals out. But for some of us, the emotions are not just occasional experiences. They are a way of living. If this is true for you, if you create your own major stress out of what, for many people, would be a minor inconvenience, you are at risk for both high blood pressure and a heart attack.

Friedman and Rosenman coined a new phrase in their book *Type A Personality.* Your deep innate personality pretty well determines how you react to the challenges of life. People with Type A personalities are demanding, time conscious, aggressive, dissatisfied and perfectionists.

Although many of us may have several of the characteristics listed above and do quite well, it takes the "big three" to make Type A extremely malignant. These three emotions are the killers: hostility, anger and frustration – a combination that allows for little joy.

If you fit the profile, it's time to "chill out." Here are a few clues. Don't take life so seriously. Avoid situations you know will deteriorate into conflict. Go ahead and strive, but do it with joy! Be exacting if you choose, but do it with humor, mostly laughing at yourself. When impatient, use this emotion as a signal to be more kind to those around you. If you feel anger, take it out with physical exercise instead of exploding or stuffing it.

You can do this with deep breathing, relaxation training, prayer, meditation, biofeedback, or systematic muscle relaxation. There are dozens of methods and books on each. Find one that fits you and use it! This will not only lower your blood pressure, but it will make you a much nicer person to be around!

OBESITY

Americans are the fattest society in the history of the world! Over 70 percent of people in the United States are overweight, and the number continues to rise. In one study, weight loss of about 10 pounds resulted in an average drop of five points in systolic pressure. "There's no question that weight loss prevents hypertension," reported Johns Hopkins' Paul Whelton.

Every pound of fat requires five miles of blood vessels to maintain it. Imagine the strain on the heart of eight pounds or 40 miles of blood vessels!

According to the Society of Actuaries, if you are 30 percent overweight, your risk of dying from heart disease compared to those with average weight is 44 percent higher for men and 34 percent higher for women.

EXERCISE

Yes, yes, yes, but get your doctor's okay first. Some people are so out of shape that they get winded getting up to change the television channel when the battery goes out in the automatic channel changer.

Your first goal is to use exercise in conjunction with weight loss. At the same time, begin to build your aerobic capacity. About 30 to 45 minutes of moderate-intensity exercise such as brisk walking, jogging, hiking, cycling or swimming is better than more exhaustive exercises.

A recent review of 40 studies concluded that people with mild hypertension can reduce both systolic and diastolic blood pressure by an average of about 10 points within three months, by performing aerobic exercise at least 20 minutes a day, three times a week.

Exercise has a fantastic additional benefit. It has long been accepted as normal that a person's blood pressure goes up with age, but that is not necessarily so. "Exercise has a unique and independent effect on preventing the age-related rise in blood pressure," says William Haskell of Stanford University. This is a real exercise bonus! It's time to get up and get moving. Pulling the plug in the bathtub and swimming against the current doesn't count!

Supplement Your Diet

AN EXPLANATION

Food supplements can be of great benefit to our health, but this philosophy runs counter to most modern conventional American medical wisdom.

We know vitamins and minerals are important because we know what happens when we don't get them. This is a big problem in advancing the science of nutrition. We work backwards from investigating diseases caused by deficiencies, instead of forward to see what extra amounts may do for our health. Therefore, our knowledge is somewhat limited because there is insufficient money available for this type of research. Huge drug companies finance much of the medical research. They then make millions on some drug developed out of the research. The problem is these companies can't make this big money by doing research on nutrients. They can't patent foods.

We hear the same old comment from the National Research Council of the National Academy of Sciences concerning taking daily vitamin and mineral supplements: "No research exists to support the practice." My answer is: "Then get busy and do the research!" Such warnings serve only to endanger the health of Americans. The suggested intakes by various government agencies do not reflect the higher amounts at which some vitamins and minerals can provide real health benefits.

Let's hear what a real health expert has to say about food supplements. Dr. Bernardine Healy is the former director of the National Institute of Health, president of the American Heart Association and has led a wide variety of White House and government advisory committees on health and science. We could go on and on with her credentials, but I want you to grasp the fact that she is a brilliant and very respected person in the medical world.

"Whatever the RDA or the medical community may recommend officially, I will tell you that increasing numbers of medical professionals are, themselves, taking supplements of these vitamins. I take supplements of calcium, the antioxidant vitamins, and a multi-vitamin. My husband and children also take vitamins," says Dr. Healy.

What is important for you to know is that some vitamins and minerals might actually prevent serious diseases such as high blood pressure. Not getting optimal nutrition for this problem should rank high alongside the risk factors of overweight, excess alcohol, a high sodium intake and all the rest.

MULTI-VITAMIN/MINERAL

The multi is really an insurance for many nutrients that may be low or missing in your diet. Are these nutrients truly missing?

Numerous studies have shown that the average American does not get all of the nutrients we need in the necessary amounts. "U.S. survey data seem to indicate that the majority of Americans do not have nutrient intakes that meet the RDAs for most vitamins and minerals," says Dr. Donna Porter, Specialist in Life Sciences at the Library of Congress, concerning a summary of the various food consumption surveys.

Note this comment from the University of Texas Lifetime Health Letter. "Though we eat enough to get fat, we frequently don't eat the right foods. More people than ever appear to be at risk of dietary deficiencies."

Food processing, extensive advertising by the huge food companies and our poor food choices are to be blamed. The multi is a good starting point for any nutrition program and should be a part of every American's daily routine.

A good multi will contain all of the vitamins with a Daily Value right at 100 percent. The exceptions are vitamins C and E. I would depend on a separate supplement for calcium and magnesium.

WATER

Water is vital to health. Drink at least eight glasses of purified clean water daily. We are made mostly of water, about 60 to 70 percent, in fact. It is a magnificent solvent and is the environment in which virtually all of our life functions are carried out.

Since water is such an excellent solvent, our water can contain much more than just H_2O. Many toxic materials can arrive from the tap into your glass via the water. We have over 66,000 synthetic chemicals in our environment. Some of these chemicals, such as compounds containing cadmium, can have bad effects on blood pressure.

CALCIUM

This vital mineral, often in short supply in our freely chosen diets, has multiple functions, some just recently discovered. Besides building strong bones and teeth, calcium can ward off osteoporosis, heart disease, some forms of cancer and help prevent, or control, high blood pressure.

"Dietary calcium intake fails to meet recommended levels in virtually all categories of Americans," was the first line in an article reporting the findings of a National Institutes of Health Consensus Conference on calcium. An analysis of the best studies available on calcium and blood pressure was reviewed. The conclusion: "These trials provide compelling evidence that hypertensive individuals may experience reductions in blood pressure when calcium intake is increased."

Here is a quick summary of their findings:

- There is a threshold of calcium intake below which high blood pressure occurs.

- The average intake of calcium in the United States is right at the threshold.

- People with high blood pressure consistently consume calcium below the threshold.

- There is no doubt at all that increasing calcium intake reduces the incidence of pregnancy-induced hypertension by more than 70 percent. Pre-eclampsia (high blood pressure, fluid retention, visible swelling, protein leaking into the urine, headache, blurred vision and nausea) was reduced by over 60 percent.

- The recommendation for pregnant women and adolescent females is 1,200 to 1,500 mg, but the average intake is only 600 to 700 mg.

For a number of reasons, high blood pressure being just one, calcium is too vital for preventive health care for you to trust only your diet for optimal intake.

In light of the research quoted previously and numerous other studies, I find it foolish not to add a calcium supplement to your diet to bring your daily calcium intake to the 1,500-milligram level.

POTASSIUM/SODIUM

Potassium participates in the electrical transmission of nerve impulses and also participates in both carbohydrate and protein metabolism. It is most important for the maintenance of normal kidney function and has a major effect on the heart and all muscles of the body.

Potassium and sodium act together to regulate the water going in and out of our cells. But to work properly, they must be in the body's preferred K-factor ratio of three.

At the beginning of the famous *Framingham Heart Study*, investigators questioned 832 healthy, middle-aged men about their diet. During a 20-year follow-up, 73 men had strokes and 24 had transient ischemic attacks (TIAs). Men who ate three or more servings of fruits and vegetables (high in potassium) daily had a 22 percent lower risk of stroke and were 50 percent less likely to die from one.

There is one danger with excess salt, regarding its effect on calcium. The more sodium you excrete, the more calcium you lose! On the average, you excrete 23 mg of calcium for every teaspoon of salt consumed. An uncompensated loss of 23 mg a day is large enough to dissolve one percent of your skeleton annually – that is 10 percent in a decade!

Excess sodium is a greater threat to your bones and eventual osteoporosis than any other nutrient. The other side of this deadly coin is the loss of calcium that we desperately need to help prevent high blood pressure. There is absolutely no good side to increased salt/sodium in your diet, and the downside can be deadly.

The best way to increase potassium is to increase consumption of fruits and vegetables. In addition to helping prevent high blood pressure, they are low in fat, high in fiber and loaded with nutrients. Perhaps there is another magic bullet in fruits and vegetables we haven't as yet identified. At any rate, routine potassium supplementation is not the best route to follow for now.

Potassium supplements are best reserved for those directly under the care of a physician. Many people taking diuretics for high blood pressure need to be on a supplement because diuretics also eliminate potassium along with sodium and water.

For now, do three things:

- Throw away the salt shaker.

- Eat more fresh vegetables and fruits. Those especially high in potassium are bananas, oranges and green leafy vegetables. Canned and frozen foods are not on the potassium preferred list. Canning and freezing change the potassium/sodium ratio in a negative way.

- If you must eat processed food, pay close attention to the label and try to buy only those foods with a K-factor of three or more.

MAGNESIUM

Study after study, from all over the world, show that daily optimal intakes of magnesium can keep blood pressure down. Magnesium can lower blood pressure all by itself. This has to do with the effect of magnesium on a kidney hormone called renin. Low levels of magnesium result in high renin levels. Renin elevates blood pressure.

Magnesium is involved in cell membrane integrity. If you are low in magnesium, the membrane becomes "leaky." This allows sodium to leak into the cell and potassium to leak out. Calcium, which should be outside the cells, also leaks into the muscle cells.

The combined result of all these leaks is that the muscles contract and the arteries become constricted. The heart must pump harder, and up goes the blood pressure.

The Daily Value (DV) for magnesium is 400 mg, but the average intake is only 268 mg. What is wrong? For one thing, the highest concentrations of magnesium are found in whole seeds such as nuts and unmilled grains. Astoundingly, more than 80 percent of the magnesium is lost by removal of the germ and outer layers of cereal grains. So much for cereal!

Green vegetables are high in magnesium, but you seldom find these in the fast-food restaurant or processed foods to which Americans seem addicted. In general, diets high in refined food, meat and man-made products tend to be low in magnesium.

You can get some magnesium from a good multi, but to be on the safe side, I would add an additional calcium/magnesium supplement.

OMEGA-3 FATTY ACIDS

All of these names apply to the same oil primarily found in cold water fish. A sister oil, also found in the fish, is docosahexaenoic acid (DHA). It occurs naturally with EPA and complements the actions of EPA. For simplicity's sake, we will just refer to it as EPA.

This oil is nature's natural "super-slick" lubricant. It is found in the membranes of cells that line the blood vessels and the membranes of the blood cells themselves. EPA has a very unique function when it comes to high blood pressure. It "lubricates" the inner walls of the vessels and makes our red blood cells more slippery.

In addition, it causes these red blood cells to be elastic and flexible, whereby they can flow more easily through tight spots. Add up these effects, and the net result is a smoother, easier flowing blood. This means the heart doesn't have to pump so hard to move the blood around and, thereby we have a lower blood pressure.

One study involved 78 patients with existing high blood pressure. Half received four grams/day of EPA and half received a placebo for only 16 weeks. In the ones taking EPA, the diastolic pressure decreased by 2.0 and the systolic by 3.8. "Fish oil has a positive effect on lipid and high blood pressure in hypertensives," said the researchers.

An adult should strive for around 1,000 to 2,000 mg of omega-3 (cold-water fish oils) a day. This equates to about three servings of cold-water, blue-skinned fish a week, such as sockeye salmon, albacore tuna, dogfish, mackerel, herring, sardines and anchovies.

If you do not like the fishy taste of fish, look for a supplement containing around 325 mg of omega-3 fatty acids (about 180 mg should be EPA). Then take two to three with each meal.

Fish vary quite a bit in their oil content. With something as serious as high blood pressure, I don't want to take any chances on coming up short.

COENZYME Q10 (CoQ10)

Scientists recently discovered that the heart contains 10 times more Coenzyme Q10 than other organs in the body. That's because your heart is the motor of your body and needs Coenzyme Q10 to provide it the energy to keep blood pumping. Levels of Coenzyme Q10 are often low in people with high blood pressure. Studies have shown that taking supplements can correct the deficiency. CoQ10 will help boost your body's ability to keep your blood pressure at healthy levels.

The mechanism by which CoQ10 brings down high blood pressure is not fully understood. It could be that CoQ10 helps your heart pump more powerfully, your circulation improves and blood flows more freely throughout your body. CoQ10 is also a powerful antioxidant, which helps make your cells healthier and less vulnerable to constriction.

CoQ10 level tends to fall dramatically with age. As foods contain very little amounts of CoQ10, the only solution is to supplement. There are many forms available: capsules, tablets, softgel in oil and hydrosoluble CoQ10 in softgel. A typical dose for high blood pressure is 60 to 90 mg of CoQ10 a day.

VITAMIN C

Vitamin C seems to be the "do-it-all" vitamin. It has been shown to reduce the risk of some cancers, help prevent heart disease, act as a powerful antioxidant, greatly increases the immune response and aid the absorption of iron. There are even more benefits. Vitamin C is involved in restoring stress hormones, aids in healing of wounds, neutralizes a number of toxic chemicals, recharges vitamin E as it is depleted and even decreases the time you have a cold and the severity of the symptoms.

Vitamin C plays a role in high blood pressure. The studies are many and most convincing. In fact, both systolic and diastolic readings are generally 5 to 10 percent lower in persons with high blood levels of vitamin C when compared to persons with low levels.

An evaluation of data from the massive United States National Health and Nutrition Examination Survey (NHANES I) shows people with lower vitamin C consumption had higher blood pressures.

Researchers at the Medical College of Georgia looked at 678 healthy men and women, 20 to 69 years of age with normal blood pressure. They discovered that those with the highest blood levels of

C had significantly lower blood pressures than those with low C levels.

Investigators at Tufts University, Boston, studied 241 Chinese Americans, some of whom had high blood pressure. The researchers found that participants with the highest blood levels of vitamin C tended to have the lowest blood pressures in the group.

The evidence has been so strong, convincing and conclusive that the USDA said people with borderline hypertension may benefit from a supplement of 1,000 mg a day. The DV of vitamin C is a mere 60 mg. I feel this is far too little for optimal health. To get 1,000 mg from diet alone is very difficult. Because of what vitamin C can do for your health, I definitely recommend a daily supplement.

B COMPLEX

The B complex came into the cardiovascular disease spotlight when it was discovered that a potentially toxic chemical from protein breakdown, called homocysteine, was responsible for some forms of heart disease. Several members of the B complex (especially folic acid) are responsible for the conversion of harmful homocysteine into methionine, an amino acid vital to our health.

This was a new finding because, in 1989, researchers thought so little of folic acid that the National Academy of Sciences (which sets the RDA) cut the recommended daily intake of the vitamin by half. New findings on the benefits of folic acid have been so astounding that the United States Food and Drug Administration will shortly be requiring that various foods be fortified with folic acid.

Before folic acid hit the news, we had to find the smoking gun. A review of 21 studies was done involving more than 1,500 patients with stroke (the end result of high blood pressure) and heart disease. They found that in 16 of these studies, patients with atherosclerosis had levels of homocysteine higher than healthier control subjects.

Further, the Harvard School of Public Health found that homocysteine promoted the growth of smooth muscle lining the walls of the arteries. This narrowing of arteries by overgrowth would obviously raise blood pressure. Finally, it was determined that three B vitamins were involved: folic acid and, to a lesser extent, B6 and B12.

Tufts University conducted an even larger study that concentrated on stroke. Individuals who consumed only moderate amounts of folic acid were about 50 percent more likely to have dangerous clogging of the carotid artery – the main vessel feeding the brain – than those who consumed large amounts of the vitamin.

The famous *Framingham Heart Study* found that a low intake of folic acid and B6 was common. For example, they discovered that 80 percent did not even consume the extremely low RDA for folic acid. All of those in this large group had high homocysteine levels. Those few who did exceed the RDA had lower homocysteine levels.

You can achieve the good folic acid number of 400 mcg and get an adequate intake of B by consuming five servings of fruits and vegetables a day. But most Americans do not eat a healthy diet with plenty of fruits and vegetables, and it is therefore wise to supplement your diet with a B complex.

These B complex vitamin supplements are inexpensive and very safe. Although ample amounts are contained in most multiple vitamins, additional B complex would be a good idea. Here is the reason: Many things widely prevalent in our American society use up the B complex at an alarming rate. Some of these are antibiotics, stress, caffeine, sugar, birth control pills, athletics, and excess alcohol. There are too many key functions of the B complex to run the risk of being even a little low.

Herbs for High Blood Pressure

GARLIC (Allium sativum)

Garlic seems to be the newly rediscovered nutritional star on the block. This amazing herb can lower blood pressure, decrease blood clotting, help prevent various cancers, block some pollutants, limit tumor growth, boost the immune system and lower cholesterol by an average of 10 percent.

Researchers combined the results of eight different studies ranging from one month to one year. They concluded that people with hypertension who took garlic supplements every day lowered their systolic pressure by an impressive eight points and their diastolic pressure by an equally impressive five points.

The bottom number, the diastolic pressure, is often considered the most critical in hypertension. In a review of 13 good studies, it was found that the average diastolic drop consistently ranged from 5 to 10 percent. Garlic combined with not smoking, weight loss, optimal diet, low salt and all of the other lifestyle factors we have mentioned concerning hypertension can have a dramatic effect on high blood pressure.

HAWTHORN (Crataegus oxyacantha)

European studies have shown that hawthorn standardized extract with its strong antioxidant properties like flavonoids can help people with high blood pressure in four ways:

- Dilates (opens) the larger blood vessels
- Increases the power of the heart

- Causes the blood to flow more smoothly
- Allows more oxygen and nutrients to reach the heart muscles

The American Herbal Product Association (AHPA) has rated hawthorn, traditionally known as "the mother of the heart," as a safe herb. If you are on heart medications such as digitalis or digoxin, be sure to consult your doctor before trying it.

GRAPE SEED EXTRACT

Grape seed extract is sourced from grape seeds. It contains OPC (oligometric proanthocyanidins), a powerful super antioxidant. Studies show it helps fight high blood pressure by:

- Strengthening capillary walls, blood vessels and veins weakened by age or disease, making them less likely to bleed, stretch, leak or burst

- Blocking the oxidation of LDL cholesterol, responsible for the buildup of arterial plague in the blood vessels

- "Reducing adrenaline stress reactions that can cause high blood pressure," says Professor Peter Rohdewald, a leading pharmaceutical researcher at the University of Munster, Germany

- Inhibiting the activity of a compound called ACE (angiotensin converting enzyme), thus helping to dilate the blood vessels and reduce the pressure being exerted by the blood against the vessels' walls

No adverse effects in humans have been reported. The grape seed extract should be standardized to contain 80 percent OPC. To maintain good vascular health, the recommended dosage is between 50 and 100 mg.

DRUGS FOR HYPERTENSION

There are about 50 drugs to treat hypertension either alone or in combination. They include:

- Diuretics
- Angiotensin converting enzyme (ACE) inhibitors
- Beta blockers
- Angiotensin II receptor blockers
- Direct vasodilators
- Calcium channel blockers
- Alpha blockers

Some of the drugs can react with others. If you are seeing more than one physician, make sure each doctor you are consulting knows exactly which medication you are taking, how much and how often. Drugs error, in one way or another, are a leading cause of hospital admission.

SUMMARY

In problems such as high blood pressure, food supplements are often necessary. They do not replace, but rather complement the other extremely important steps you must take to help prevent high blood pressure. These few healthy lifestyle changes we have mentioned, including the supplements and herbs, can possibly allow you to get off medication or at least have your medication reduced.

Many people are quite willing to take the food supplements, but are very reluctant to make the necessary lifestyle changes which enhance the actions of the supplements. The biggest problem all health providers encounter is patient compliance. It's just easier to take a drug with all of its side effects than to make some healthy changes.

Please do not be one of these people. Have the determination to change your habits as you travel along the road of life. Change your destination towards optimal health and enjoyment rather than a miserable existence. Health is not a place where you arrive. It is a daily trip made up of numerous choices. Have the courage to make the right choices; it is well worth the effort!

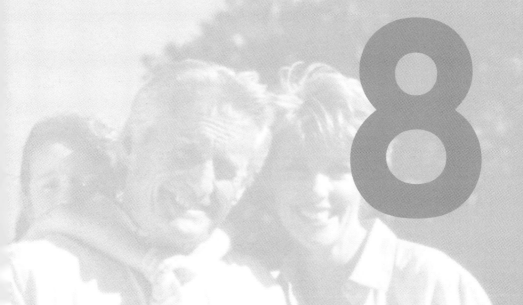

8

IN CLOSING

Taking Charge of Your CVD

Taking Charge of Your CVD

8

According to the American Heart Association's heart disease and stroke statistics 2007 update, the cost of CVD in the United States for 2006 is estimated at US$403.1 billion. Yet, while the direct and indirect costs of CVD are staggering, figures can never tell the whole story. No one can begin to quantify the suffering experienced by even one victim of CVD and his or her loved ones.

CVD victims have to cope for the rest of their lives with diminished capacities, paralysis, brain damage, kidney failure and a host of other physical, mental, and emotional difficulties. Many who have suffered a heart attack or stroke live in continual fear of having another. In fact, persons who survive an initial heart attack are five times more likely to die within the next five years than persons with no history of heart disease.

CVD is not an inevitable result of aging. You can take many preventive measures to arrest the "silent killers within" you from damaging your cardiovascular health. The American Heart Association in one of its numerous publications aptly states: "A major reduction in heart attack and heart death can be achieved only by prevention of heart attacks, not from the treatment of established heart disease. Almost half of all attack deaths occur with the first heart attack and before treatment can be started. Therefore, prevention is a must."

Some risk factors for cardiovascular health cannot be changed. Yet other risk factors can be changed. Therefore, I urge you to seek and identify your own risks from the information provided in this book, and take the necessary steps now to change your current lifestyle by discarding what is bad and practicing what is good. Hopefully, we can keep the "silent killers" within you at bay, the common sense way. I wish you the best of health!

161

BIBLIOGRAPHY

Acheson, R. Williams, "Does consumption of fruit and vegetables protect against stroke?" *The Lancet*, 1993.

Agarwal RC, et al., "Clinical trial of gugulipid – a new hypolipidemic agent of plant origin in primary hyper-lipidemia." *Indian J. Med. Res.* 1986 Dec; 84: 626-34.

Altura, B. and Altura, B., "Cardiovascular risk factors and magnesium: relationships to atherosclerosis, ischemic heart disease, and hypertension." *Magnesium Trace Element: A Review*, 1993.

American Diabetes Association and National Institute of Diabetes, Digestive and Kidney Diseases. 2002. "The prevention or delay of type 2 diabetes." *Diabetes Care* 25 (4): 1-8.

Ames. B., "Oxidants, antioxidants, and degenerative diseases of aging." *Proceedings of National Academy of Sciences*, 90(17): 7915-22, 1993.

Anderson, D. M., Castelli, W.P. and Levy, D., "Cholesterol and mortality: 30 years of follow-up from the Framingham Study." *Journal of the American Medical Association*, 257:2176-80, 1987.

Anderson, RA., "Chromium, Glucose Tolerance and Diabetes." *Biol Trace Elements Res* 32: 19-24, 1992.

Anderson, RA., "Potential antioxidant effects of zinc and chromium supplementation in type 2 diabetes mellitus." *Journal of the American College of Nutrition* 2002: 20:212-18.

Anderson, RA., "Review: Chromium, glucose intolerance and diabetes." *Journal of the American College of Nutrition* 17:548-55, 1998.

"B makes the grade." *Consumer Reports on Health*, June 1995.

Bahorum, T.B Gressier, F. Trotin et al., "Oxygen Species Scavenging Activity of Phenolic Extracts from Hawthorn Fresh Plant Organs & Pharmaceutical Preparation". 46:11 (Nov 1996): 1086-89.

Bairati, I., et al., "Effects of a fish oil supplement on blood pressure and serum lipids in patients treated for coronary artery disease." *Canadian Journal of Cardiology*, Jan./Feb. 1992.

Baskaran K, Kizar Ahamaht B et al., "Anti-diabetic effect of a leaf extract from Gymnema sylvestre in non-insulin dependent diabetes mellitus patients." *J. Ethnopharmacol* 1990 Oct: 30(3): 295-300.

Beebe, C., "Eating healthy, eating smart." *Diabetes Forecast*, Dec. 1994.

Bendich, et al., "The health effects of vitamin C supplementation: A review." *Journal of the American College of Nutrition.* 1955: 14:124-36.

Benjamin, Stephanie M., PhD and Rodolfo Valdez, PhD, et al. 2003, "Estimated number of adults with pre-diabetes in the US in 2000: Opportunities for prevention." *Diabetes Care* 26:6456-649.

Blake, G., "Control of type II diabetes." *Postgraduate Medicine*, Nov. 1992.

Brand JC et al., "A low glycemic index foods improve long-term glycemic control in NIDDM." *Diabetes Care* 1991; 14: 95-101.

Brody J., *Jane Brody's Good Food Book.* Bantam Books, 1987.

Brody, J., "Type 2 diabetes is an increasingly common killer that many patients fail to take seriously." *New York Times,* Nov. 1995.

Brown, W., "Lipoprotein disorders in diabetes mellitus." *Med Clin North Am,* Jan. 1994.

Bucher, H., Cook, R. and Guyatt, G. et al., "Effects of dietary calcium supplementation on blood pressure: a meta-analysis of randomized controlled trials." *Journal of the American Medical Association,* 1996.

Caroll, K., "Review of clinical studies on cholesterol-lowering response to soy protein." *Journal of the American Dietetic Association,* 91:820-87,1991.

Carper, J., *The Good Pharmacy Guide to Good Eating.* Bantam Books, 1991.

Carter, Jean, *"Miracle Cures."* Thorsons, 1997.

Chausmer A., "A review: Zinc, insulin and diabetes." *Journal of the American College of Nutrition.* 17: 109-115, 1998.

Cooper, K., *The Aerobics Program for Total Well-Being.* Bantam Books, 1982. Also, Cooper K. and Cooper, M., *The New Aerobics for Women.* Rev. ed. Bantam Books, 1988.

"Diabetes: Living successfully with a lifelong challenge." *Mayo Clinic Health Letter* (Medical Essay), Jun. 1992.

Digiesi V, et al., "Coenzyme Q10 is essential hypertension." *Mol Aspects Med 15 (Suppl).* 5257-5263, 1994.

Dwyer, J. T., "Health aspects of vegetarian diets." *American Journal of Clinical Nutrition,* 48 (3 suppl.): 712-38, 1988.

Estrada DE, et al., "Stimulation of glucose uptake by the natural coenzyme alpha lipoic acid." *Diabetes* 45: 1798-804, 1996.

"Exercise for blood pressure reduction." *Harvard Heart Letter,* April 1994. Also see: *Circulation,* Dec. 1993.

"Fifth Report Of The Joint National Committee On Detection, Evaluation And Treatment Of High Blood Pressure." National Institutes of Health. NIH publication No. 93-1088, 1992.

"Fish prevent strokes by fifty percent." *HealthNews,* April 6, 1996. See also: *Archives of Internal Medicine,* Mar. 1996.

Folkers, K. "Heart failure is a dominant deficiency of Coenzyme Q10 and challenges for future clinical research on CoQ10." *Clinical Investigator* 1993: 71(Suppl): S51-54.

Folkers, K. Yamamura Y (eds) Elsevier/North-Holland Biomedical Press Amsterdam, 1977, pp. 251-265.

Franz, M., "The nutrition intervention study." *Diabetes Self-Management,* May/June 1995.

"Garlic." *Nutrition Action Healthletter,* July/Aug. 1995.

Gaziano, J., "The role of beta-carotene in the prevention of cardiovascular disease." *Annals of the New York Academy of Sciences,* 691: 148-55. 1993.

Gerrits, P. and Tsalikian, E., "Diabetes and fructose metabolism." *Am J Clin Nutr,* Nov. 1993.

Golub, C., "Diabetes: promising new therapies for an age-old disease." *Environmental Nutrition,* Mar. 1996.

Greenberg, S., "Coenzyme Q10: a new drug for cardiovascular disease." *Journal of Clinical Pharmacology* 1990:30(7): 596-608.

Gretchen Becker, *Pre-diabetes: What you need to know to keep diabetes away.* Marlowe and Company N.Y. 15.1.05.

Griffin, G. and Castelli, W., *How To Lower Your Cholesterol and Beat the Odds of a Heart Attack.* Fisher Books, 1993.

Haire-Joshu, D. Ziff, S., "Where there's smoke there's complication." *Diabetes Forecast,* Mar. 1994.

Harman, D. 1956. "Aging: A theory based on free radical and radiation chemistry." *Journal of Gerontology* 11:298 300.

Haskell, W., Spiller, G., Jensen, C., Ellis, B. and Gates, J., "Role of water-soluble dietary fiber in the management of elevated plasma cholesterol in healthy subjects." *American Journal of Cardiology,* 69: 433-9, 1992.

Henry, R., "Glucose control and insulin resistance in non-insulin-dependent diabetes mellitus." *Ann Intern Med,* Jan.1996.

"High blood pressure: a complete guide to treatment." *Consumer reports on Health,* May 1995.

Hobbs C and Foster S. "Hawthorn-Alternative Review". *Herbalgram* 22 (1990): 19-33.

Hoffman, R., "Antioxidants and the prevention of coronary heart disease." *Archives of Internal Medicines,* 155(3): 241-46, 1995.

"Hypertension: mild no more." *Harvard Health Letter,* March 1993.

"Important news on diabetes." *Health after 50 (Johns Hopkins Medical Letter),* Feb. 1996.

Jacques, P., "Effects of vitamin C on high density lipoprotein, cholesterol and blood pressure." *Journal of the American College of Nutrition,* 62: 252-55, 1992.

Jensen, C., Spiller, G., Gates, J., Miller, A. and Whittman J., "The effect of acacia gum and water-soluble dietary fiber mixture on blood lipids in humans." *Journal of the American College of Nutrition,* 12:147-54, 1993.

Jialal, I., "The effect of a-tocopherol supplementation on LDL oxidation and vitamin E: a dose response study." *Atherosclerosis, Thrombosis and Vascular Biology,* 15(2): 190-198, 1995.

Kerman, A., "Could you lower your blood pressure without drugs?" *Executive Health's Good Health Report,* Dec. 1993.

Kerman, A., The H.A.R.T. Program: Lowering Blood Pressure Without Drugs. *Harper Perennial,* 1993.

Klein, R. and Klein, B., "Relation of glycemic control to diabetic microvascular complication in diabetes mellitus." *Ann Inter Med*, Jan. 1996.

Krakoff, L., "Even calm relaxed people have high blood pressure." *Executive Health's Good Health Report*, April 1996.

Krakoff, L., *Management of the Hypertensive Patient*. Churchill Livingston Publishers, 1995.

Kochar, M. and Kalluru, V., "Hypertension in the diabetic patient." *Postgraduate Medicine*, Nov. 1994.

Lagrue, G., "A study of the effects of procyanidol oligomers on capillary resistance in hypertension and in certain nephropathies." *Sem. Hop* 57 (33-36): 399-401, 198.

Lands, W., "Biochemistry and physiology of n-3 fatty acids" *FASEB Journal*, 6: 2530-36,1992.

Langford, H., "Non-pharmacological therapy of hypertension: commentary on diet and blood pressure." *Hypertension*, 1989.

Langsjoen, P., et al., "Usefulness of coenzyme Q10 in clinical cardiology: long term study." *Molecular Aspects Medicine* 15 (Suppl. PS): 165-175, 1994.

Langsjoen, P.H. and Folkers, Karl. "Treatment of hypetrophic cardiomyopathy with Coenzyme Q10." *Molecular Aspects of Medicine* Vol.18 Suppl.:S145-151, 1997.

Lanthony P, Cosson JP., "The course of colour vision in early diabetic retinopathy treated with ginkgo biloba extract. A preliminary double-blind versus placebo study." *J French Opthalmol* 1988; 11(10): 671-4.

Leatherdale BA, Panesar RK, Singh G, et al., "Improvement of glucose tolerance due to Momordica charanti (Karela)." *British Medical Journal (Clinin Res Ed)* 282:1823-1824, 1981.

Packer, L., PhD, *The Antioxidant Miracle*. John Wiley and Sons, Inc. 1999.

Liebman, B., "One nation under pressure." *Nutrition Action Healthletter*, Aug. 1995. See also *Hypertension* 25: 305, 1995; *Annals of Epidemiology* 5: 108, 1995; and *Journal of the American Medical Association* 273: 11-13, 1995.

Liebman, B., "The salt shake out." *Nutrition Action Healthletter*, March 1994.

Madar Z, et al. "Glucose lowering effect of fenugreek in non-insulin dependent diabetics." *European Journal of Clinical Nutrition* 42: 51-54, 1998.

Madar Z, Abel R, Samish S, Arad J., "Glucose lowering effect of fenugreek in non-insulin dependent diabetes." *Eur J Clin Nutr* 1988 Jan; 4211: 51-4.

Manson, J., "Antioxidants and cardiovascular disease: a review." *Journal of the American College of Nutrition*, 12(4): 426-32, August 1993.

McCarron, D. and Hatton, D., "Dietary calcium and lower blood pressure, we can all benefit." *Journal of the American Medical Association*, April 1996. Also see *Journal of the American Medical Association*, April 3, 1996.

McKeigue PM., "Ethnic variations in insulin

resistance and glucose tolerance, in *Insulin Resistance: The Metabolic Syndrome X*." 19-34, 1999.

McLaughlin T, Abassi F, et al., "Relationship between insulin resistance, weight loss, and coronary heart disease in healthy, obese women." *Metabolism* 7:795-800, 2001.

Mason, Michael, "The Insulin Threat: Carbohydrates and your heart." *Health* 3/00.

Mindell, E., *Earl Mindell's Soy Miracle*. Fireside. 1995.

Murphy, R., "Management of diabetic retinopathy." *American Family Physician*, Mar. 1995.

Nathan, D., "The pathophysiology of diabetic complication: How much does the glucose hypothesis explain?" *Ann Intern Med*, Jan. 1996.

National Diabetes Information Clearinghouse 2004. "Am I at risk for type 2 diabetes? Taking steps to lower the risk of getting diabetes." *National Institute of Health*. April.

Niaz, MA, and Chosh, S., "Hypolipidemic and antioxidant effects of Commiphora mukul (gugulipid) as an adjunct to dietary therapy in patients with hypercholesterolmia." *Cardiovascular Drugs and Therapeutics* (1994) 8: 659-664.

Nityanand S., J. Srivastava JS and O. Asthana, "Clinical Trials with gugulipid. A New Hypolipidemic Agent." *J Assoc. Physicians India* 37: 5 (May 1989): 323-28.

"Nutrition recommendations and principles for people with diabetes mellitus." *Journal of the American Dietetic Association*, May 1994.

O'Brien, J., "The first world congress on the health significance of garlic and garlic constituents." *Trends in food science and Technology*, Dec. 1990.

Ornish, D., *Reversing Heart Disease*. Ballantine Books, 1990.

Packer, et al., "Review: Alpha lipoic acid as a biological antioxidant." *Free Radicals in Biology and Medicine*.

Packer, L., "Vitamin E and diabetes mellitus." *Diabetes and Stoffwechsel* 1997: 6:2-3.

Palca, J., "Vitamin C gets a little respect." *Science*, Oct. 1991.

Paolisso, "Daily magnesium supplements improve glucose handling in elderly subjects." *American Journal of Clinical Nutrition*, 55 (1992), 1161-1167.

Pastors, J., et. al., "Psyllium fiber reduces rise in postprandial glucose and insulin concentrations in patients with non-insulin-dependent diabetes." *Am J Clin Nutr*, Jun. 1991.

Popping S. et al., Effect of a Hawthorn extract on contraction and energy turnover of isolated rat. *Cadiummyongtes Arzneimittelforschung Drug Res* 45:1157-1661, 1995.

"Pressing garlic for possible health benefits." *Tufts University Diet and Nutrition Letter*, 12(7): 3, September 1994.

Reaven, G.M., Chen, T.D.I., Jeppesen, J., Maheux, P., Krauss, R.M., "Insulin resistance and hyper-insulinemia in individuals with small, dense, low density lipoprotein particles." *Journal of Clinical Investigation.*

Reaven GM, Storm TK, Fox B, *Syndrome X The Silent Killer.* Simon and Schuster, 2000.

Rimm, et al., "Vitamin E consumption and the risk of coronary heart disease in men." 1993: 328 (20): 1450-56.

Rodale, J. *The Hawthorn Berry for the heart.* Emmacus: Rodale Press, 1971.

Rubin, R., "Rising to the challenge of tight control." *Diabetes Self-Management,* Jan./Feb. 1995.

Sacks, F., "Dietary Fats and blood pressure: a critical review of the evidence." *Nutrition Reviews,* 1989.

Sacks, F. "Therapy to molecular mechanisms." *Annals of the New York Academy of Sciences* 676: 188-201, 1993.

Savage, P., "Cardiovascular complication of diabetes mellitus: What we know and what we need to know about their prevention." *Ann Intern Med,* Jan. 1996.

Schulz V. et al., *Rational phytotherapy.* New York: Springer-Verlap 1998: 91-95.

Shanmugasundaram ERB, et al. "Use of Gymnema sylvestre leaf extract in the control of blood glucose in insulin dependent diabetes mellitus." *Journal Ethnopharmacol* 30: 281-294, 1990.

Sharma RD, Raghuram TC, et al., "Effect of fenugreek seeds on blood glucose and serum lipids in type 1 diabetes." *European Journal of Clinical Nutrition* 44:301-306, 1990.

Sharma RD, Raghuram TC, Rao NS., "Effect of fenugreek on blood glucose and serum lipids in type 1 diabetes." *European Journal of Clinical Nutrition* 44: 300–5, 1990.

Silagy, C., "Garlic as a lipid lowering agent-a meta-analysis." *Journal of the Royal College of Physicians.* London 28 (1):39-45, 1994.

Sinatra ST., "Refractory congestive heart failure successfully managed with high dose coenzyme Q10 administration." *Molecular Aspects Medicine* 18 (supp): s299-s305, 199.

Slavin, J., "Nutritional benefits of soy protein and soy fiber." *Journal of the American Dietetic Association,* 91: 816-19, 1991.

Stampfer, M., "Homocysteine and marginal vitamin deficiency: the importance of adequate vitamin intake:" *Editorial. Journal of the American Medical Association,* 270(22): 2726, 1993.

Stampfer, M., "Vitamin E consumption and the risk of coronary disease in women." *New England Journal of Medicine,* 328: 1444-49, 1993.

Street D., "Serum antioxidants and myocardial infarction." *Circulation,* 90: 1154-19, 1994.

"Stress, hypertension and length of life." *Harvard Heart Letter,* April 1994. Also see: *British Medical Journal,* October 30, 1993.

"Stress, salt and blood pressure." *Wellness Letter,* April 1993.

"Study pressures doctors to treat hypertensive seniors." *People's Medical Society,* Dec.1995.

"Support for cardiovascular benefits of vitamin C." *Harvard Heart Letter,* Dec. 1995. Also: *British Medical Journal,* June 17, 1995.

Taunton, J. and McCargar, "Managing activity in patient who have diabetes." *Physician and Sportsmedecine,* Mar. 1995.

McCully, K., *The Homocysteine Revolution* (Keats Publishing 1997).

"Third Report of the NCEP Expert Panel on Detection, Evaluation, and Treatment of High Blood Cholesterol in Adults," also known as Adult Treatment Panel (ATP)III *Journal of the American Medical Association,* May 16, 2001.

Thomas T. and Londeree, B., "Energy cost during prolonged walking vs. jogging exercise." *The Physician and Sports*

Medicine 17: 93-102, 1989.

"TIAs: heeding an early warning for stroke." *Health after 50,* Dec. 1994.

Tobian L., "Potassium and Sodium in hypertension." *Journal of Hypertension,* 1998.

Toft, I., et al., "Effects of n-3 polyunsaturated fatty acids on glucose homeostasis and blood pressure in essential hypertension." *Annals of Internal Medicine,* 1995.

Vegetarian – live longer. *British Medical Journal,* 308: 1667-771, 1994.

"Vitamins and Heart Disease: A Homocysteine Connection?" *Harvard Heart Letter,* Oct. 1994.

Weihmayr, T. and E Ernst., "Therapeutic Effectiveness of Crataegus" *Frotschritte de medizu* 114: 1-2 (20 Jan. 1996): 27-29.

Winter, R., *Medicines In Food.* Crown Publishing, 1995.

GLOSSARY

Aneurysm: A localized "ballooning-out" of the wall of a blood vessel. The increased pressure in the blood vessel coupled with a weakened wall results in aneurysm. An aneurysm may rupture and cause fatal hemorrhages.

Angina: A condition in which the heart muscles receive an insufficient blood supply, resulting in chest pain in the left arm and shoulder. The chest pain of angina is typically severe and crushing.

Artery: A large blood vessel that carries blood from the heart to other parts of the body. Arteries are thicker and have walls that are stronger and more elastic than the walls of veins.

Atherosclerosis: A process of progressive clogging, narrowing and hardening of the walls of the body's large arteries and medium-sized blood vessels as a result of fat deposits on their inner lining. Atherosclerosis is the root cause of most cardiovascular disease.

Beta cell: A type of cell in the pancreas that makes and releases insulin to control the level of glucose (sugar) in the blood. Within the pancreas, the beta cells are located in areas called the *Isles of Langerhans*.

Blood glucose: The main sugar that the body makes from the food in the diet. Glucose is the major source of energy for living cells and is carried to each cell through the bloodstream. Cells cannot use glucose without the help of insulin.

Blood glucose meter: A machine that helps test how much glucose (sugar) is in the blood.

Body Mass Index (BMI): A measure used to evaluate body weight relative to a person's height. BMI is used to find out if a person is underweight, normal weight, overweight or obese. To calculate your BMI, divide your weight by your height squared.

Blood pressure: Pressure in the arteries is our blood pressure. Blood pressure is read as two numbers: systolic and diastolic. Systolic pressure is generated when your heart muscle contracts and forcefully sends the blood through the arteries. The diastolic pressure is the remaining pressure in the arteries while the heart is refilling and getting ready to beat again. If your systolic pressure is 120 and your diastolic is 80, it would be written as 120/80. Elevation of blood pressure is called "hypertension."

Blood vessels: Tubes that carry blood to and from all parts of the body. The three main types of blood vessels are arteries, veins, and capillaries.

Cataract: Clouding of the lens of the eye. In people with diabetes, this condition is sometimes referred to as "sugar cataract."

Cardiovascular disease: Disease of the heart and blood vessels (arteries, veins, and capillaries).

Cholesterol: An odorless, white, powdery fatty substance similar to fat produced by the liver and found in the blood. It is also found in some foods. Cholesterol is used by the body to make hormones and build cell walls. An elevated level of blood cholesterol is a major cause of coronary heart disease.

Coma: A sleep-like state in which a person is not conscious. This could be caused by hyperglycemia (high blood glucose) or hypoglycemia (low blood glucose) in people with diabetes.

Congestive heart failure: Loss of the heart's pumping power, which causes fluids to collect in the body, especially in the feet and lungs. Congestive heart failure often develops gradually over several years, although it also can happen suddenly.

Coronary heart disease: This disease is caused by narrowing of the arteries that supply blood to the heart mainly due to cholesterol deposits in the artery walls. If the blood supply is cut off, the result is a heart attack.

Diabetes: Diabetes results when our body cannot use blood glucose as energy because of having too little insulin or being unable to use insulin. There are two major forms of diabetes. In type 1 diabetes the pancreas no longer makes insulin and therefore blood glucose cannot enter the cells to be used for energy. In type 2 diabetes, either the pancreas does not make enough insulin or the body is unable to use insulin correctly.

Diabetic neuropathy: A family of nerve disorders caused by diabetes. Diabetic neuropathies cause numbness and sometimes pain and weakness in the hands, arms, feet, and legs.

Diabetic retinopathy: A common complication of diabetes affecting the small blood vessels in the retina. If untreated, it may lead to blindness.

Fasting blood glucose test: A method of checking a person's blood glucose level after an overnight fast. This test is used to diagnose pre-diabetes and diabetes. It is also used to monitor people with diabetes.

Gangrene: The death of body tissue, most often caused by a lack of blood flow and infection. It can lead to amputation.

Gestational diabetes mellitus (GDM): A type of diabetes mellitus that develops only during pregnancy and usually disappears upon delivery, but increases the risk that the mother will develop diabetes later.

Glaucoma: An eye disease associated with increased pressure within the eye. Glaucoma can damage the optic nerve and cause loss of vision and blindness.

Glucose: Glucose is the principal sugar the body makes. It is the body's main source of energy. The body makes glucose from proteins, fats and carbohydrates. Glucose is carried to each cell through the bloodstream.

Glucose tolerance test: A blood test done to find out how your body can handle excess sugar after drinking a high dose of a glucose drink. This is another test for diabetes.

Glycemic index: A ranking of how fast 50 grams of a carbohydrate-containing food is converted into glucose and enters the bloodstream. Pure glucose or white bread has a ranking of a 100 on the GI and all other carbohydrates are ranked in relation to glucose.

Glycemic load: The glycemic load of a food is calculated by multiplying the glycemic index by the actual number of grams of carbohydrate eaten in a meal and dividing the total by 100.

Heart attack: A heart attack occurs from the blockage in one of the coronary arteries due to atherosclerosis. The blockage stops the blood supply to the heart muscle. Without the necessary oxygen that comes in the blood, the part affected becomes damaged. Depending upon the severity of the damage, disability or death can result.

HDL cholesterol: High-density lipoprotein (HDL), the "good" cholesterol found in the blood that takes extra cholesterol from the bloodstream to the liver for removal.

HbA1C test: This test offers you a picture of how high your blood glucose has been for the last three months.

Hyperglycemia: A higher-than-normal amount of glucose in the blood, a sign that diabetes is out of control.

Hypoglycemia: Less than normal amount of glucose in the blood, popularly called low blood sugar.

Hyperinsulinemia: A condition in which the level of insulin in the blood is higher than normal.

Hyperlipidemia: Higher than normal fat and cholesterol levels in the blood.

Hypotension: Low blood pressure or a sudden drop in blood pressure. A person rising quickly from a sitting or reclining position may have a sudden fall in blood pressure, causing dizziness or fainting.

Insulin: A natural hormone made by the pancreas that controls the level of the sugar glucose in the blood. Insulin permits cells to use glucose for energy. Cells cannot utilize glucose without insulin.

Insulin receptors: Areas on the outer part of a cell that allow the cell to bind with insulin in the blood. When the cell and insulin bind, the cell can take glucose from the blood and use it for energy.

Insulin resistance: A condition in which the body cells refuse to let insulin shuttle glucose into it. This resistance by the cells causes glucose to remain high in the bloodstream.

Kidney failure: A chronic condition in which the body retains fluid and harmful wastes build up because the kidneys no longer work properly.

LDL cholesterol: Low-density lipoprotein (LDL), a fat found in the blood, takes cholesterol around the body to where it is needed for cell repair and also deposits it on the inside of artery walls. It is often called "bad" cholesterol.

Lipid: A term for fat in the body. Lipids can be broken down by the body and used for energy.

Mg/dL: Milligrams per deciliter. The units used by Americans when measuring blood glucose and lipid levels. European countries use SI units (mmol/L).

Pre-diabetes: A condition in which blood glucose levels are higher than normal but are not high enough to be classified as diabetes. People with pre-diabetes are at increased risk for developing type 2 diabetes and for heart disease and stroke. Other names for pre-diabetes are impaired glucose tolerance and impaired fasting glucose.

Pre-prandial blood glucose: The blood glucose level taken before eating.

Stroke: The death of brain cells due to a lack of oxygen when the blood flow to the brain is impaired by blockage or rupture of an artery to the brain. This may cause loss of ability to speak or to move parts of the body.

Triglyceride: The storage form of fat in the body. High triglyceride levels may occur when diabetes is out of control.

Vein: A blood vessel that carries blood to the heart.